Healthy Kids Don't Eat Poison APPLES

LISA HEATHER TORBERT

ISBN: 1533422664
ISBN 13: 9781533422668
Cover Artist: Aekyung Maria Ruffin
Author Photo: David Wolanski
Proofreaders
Krystal Gil
Wendy Wittmayer-Davis
Michelle Gillott
Nan Weaver
Ann Gravatt
Mike McCoy

This book is dedicated to all of my grandkids; the loves of my life, the apples of my eye!

Casher William Schellinger (front cover)
John Joseph Quinn
Chloe Noelle Quinn
Abbey Nichole Quinn
Morgan Elizabeth Ramsey
Seth Hunter Ramsey
Grandmom Spells Love

Grandmom's have fun without the worry
Raising is for parents, we get quality without the hurry
Angels go back home, the special time feels like heaven
No getting up, no waiting up, no 24/seven
Doing things out of pure love, giving endlessly till we tire
Money's not an issue, we give them what they desire
Opening our hearts, magical moments, getting wild
Memories that last forever, having fun with our grandchild

My prayers go out to all the children of the world, especially those that are suffering from one of the seven childhood diseases. After reading this book, may parents use it like a handbook, to reference many of the remedies and make changes to bring good health to your little bundles of joy, no matter how old they are.

My prayers go out to all of the doctors, researchers, teachers and parents. May we unite together and start to change our vision; from medications to prevention, from junk food to home cooked organic food, from chemical cleaners to holistic ones, from killing the already diseased bodies with chemicals to boosting the immune system with antioxidants, from greed to cures!

Disclaimer: This book contains general information about medical treatments and holistic approaches using natural remedies. Do not rely on the information in this book as an alternative to medical advice from your doctor or other professional healthcare providers. Always consult your doctor or health care provider for any questions, changes in your health, or medical conditions. Never delay seeking treatment or disregard medical advice. Never discontinue medical treatment including medications without your doctor's advice. If you want to try some of these recommended holistic treatments, always consult with your doctor first. Most doctors are compliant and can work with your child to integrate holistic practices with your current treatments.

TABLE OF CONTENTS

Chapter 1 *"Mirror, Mirror,"* Who is the Sickest of them All? Our Kids ····· 1
Chapter 2 *"Who's Afraid of the Big Bad Wolf"* – Toxins in Newborns ······· 7
Chapter 3 *"Strong to the Finish, Cause I Eat my Spinach"* – What to Eat? ···· 12
Chapter 4 *"Monsters Inc."* ADHD, Autism, & All Kids ··············· 29
Chapter 5 *"Saving Good Health from Bad Science"* – Autism ············ 71
Chapter 6 *"I Can't Huff or Puff or Blow your House Down"* Asthma ········ 87
Chapter 7 *"Khemical Kids"* – Medications and Vaccinations ··········· 97
Chapter 8 *"Honey, I Blew Up the Kids"* Fat Kids & Diabetes ··········· 122
Chapter 9 *"Twinkle Twinkle"* – Too Much Technology ················128
Chapter 10 *"Angry Birds"* Negative Effects from TV, Movies, Games······143
Chapter 11 *"Goosebumps"* Relaxation for Kids ····················149
Chapter 12 *"How to Train Your Dragon"* – Discipline ················161
Chapter 13 *"And on this Farm He Had a Cow"* Breastfeeding, Formula, Milk····178
Chapter 14 *"Do You Know the Muffin Man?"* White Flour & Sugar ······· 192
Chapter 15 *"I'm a Little Teapot"* - Healthy Drinks for Kids ··········· 203
Chapter 16 *"Cloudy With a Chance of Meatballs"* Serving Poison on Your Plate ··213
Chapter 17 *"Finding Nemo"* Fish Tails and Tales ···················219
Chapter 18 *"Rub a Dub Dub"* Cleaning Products ················· 224
Chapter 19 *"SpongeBob SquarePants"* Toxic Diapers ················242
Chapter 20 *"Tangled"* Hair and Skin Care Products ················ 252
Chapter 21 *"Sleeping Beauty"* How to Get to Sleep and Stay There ······ 264
Chapter 22 *"Toy Story"* – Safety, Learning, Bad Plastic ·············· 272
Chapter 23 *"Beauty and the Beast"* Hormone Balance················ 280
Chapter 24 *"Rain Rain Go Away"* Children's Addiction & Depression···· 287
Chapter 25 *"The Wonderful World of Ahhh"* Detoxing ··············· 292
Lisa Heather Torbert - Biography ··························· 303
Bibliography································· 305

1

"MIRROR, MIRROR," WHO IS THE SICKEST OF THEM ALL? OUR KIDS

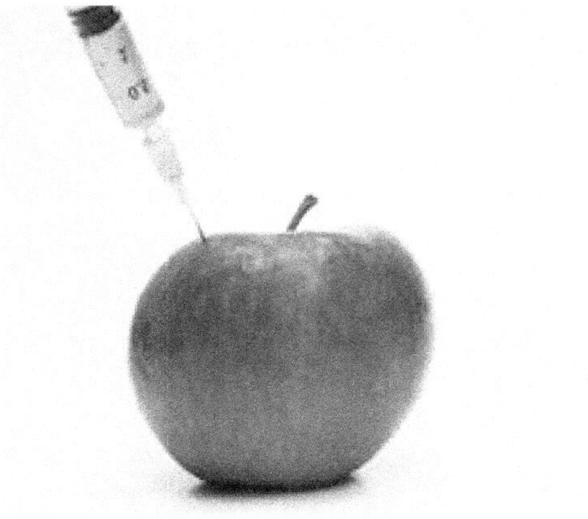

Once upon a time, there were beautiful newborn babies who were pure, healthy and happy. Then evil crept into their lives and no magic could protect them from these toxins. The leader of the Kingdom cast an evil spell allowing the poisonous chemicals to be spread throughout the land; tricking parents into thinking everything was healthy. The parents cleaned their castles with chemicals and lathered their kids with more toxics. They did not know better and fed their kids foods sprayed with the invisible poisons. One day they took their children to the doctor they trusted for a hefty shot of toxins, telling them they were the most potent weapon to protect them and keep them safe. On the way home, the parents stopped at the market to buy some beautiful shiny red apples, unbeknown that they too were disguised with more sprayed toxins. When they bit into the apples, the children became very sick. Soon they were no longer **Happy**, but had become **Sneezy**, **Grumpy, Bashful and Sleepy**. The **Doc** told the parents their kids had become **Dopey**. "No kiss will save our sleeping beauties from these poison apples." But you as parents now hold the magic wand that can break the spell holding our children hostage. It is time to turn our creepy crawly caterpillars into beautiful butterflies whose wings will transport us to another level of health.

The First 7 Days of Life – A Dwarf in Development

"Hi Ho…Hi Ho"…it's home from the hospital we go! We wrap our little prince or princess in Snow White bleached blankets and bring them home to our castles we have cleaned like Cinderella, scrubbing with our toxic cleaning products, giving ourselves and baby a whiff of chemicals before they are even born. Some of us decide to feed our babies formula, which is saturated with corn syrup and chemicals. We expose them to toxins used in conventional cleaners, wash and dry their clothes in chemicals, slather them in chemical lotions and creams, bathe them with toxic soaps and shampoos and sprinkle their developing lungs with baby powder dust, "not pixie approved." If we bottle feed, we let them suck on BPA plastic nipples and pacifiers. Our Sleeping Beauties lie on chemically treated mattresses, and breathe its' toxic fumes. When they get a little older, we feed them foods treated with pesticides, and milk and meats loaded with antibiotics and hormones. With this tornado of toxins invading our young children today, we need a magical land of Oz to help us reduce the increasing odds for the 7 deadly diseases: Autism, ADHD, ADD, Asthma, SIDs, Diabetes and Obesity. "There's no place like healthy". We rack our **brains** to understand, muster up the **courage** to help them heal and we open up our **hearts** to love them unconditionally.

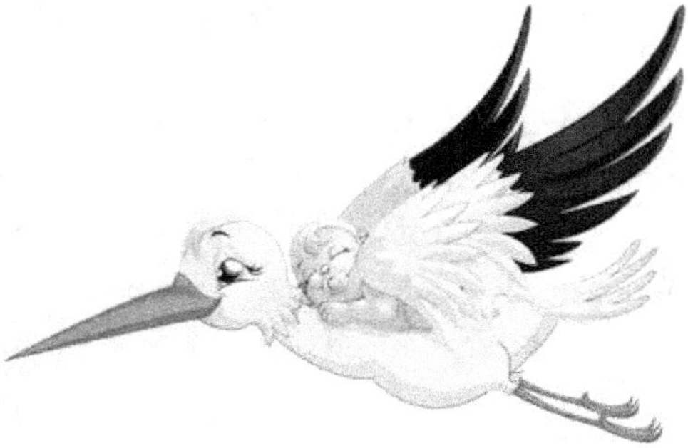

Most of us have seen that famous scene in the Disney movie "Dumbo" where the stork delivers baby to his mommy. Wouldn't it be nice if it were that easy to have a healthy baby? Did you know storks are known for their parental dedication? They will continue to feed and care for their young even after they are able to fly. Some of us will have to do that out of necessity because our children are so sick today.

Today's statistics in the United States paints a picture with realism:

1 out of every 3 kids are overweight or obese
1 out of every 10 kids have ADHD/ADD
1 out of every 10 kids have asthma
1 out of every 63 kids have autism (1 in every 49 Boys)

Mommy's House of Gingerbread

The trouble with toxins started long before our babies even enter their 9-month home. Deep in our bellies, our baby's home is constructed of gingerbread, cookies and candy. If mommy eats fast food, processed food, and the "evil whites" (sugar, flour, rice) before ever becoming pregnant, then she already is carrying a toxic load, which will be part of the nourishment our "little bundles of joy" will live on.

For those of you who are planning to have a baby, your first step is to clean up the toxicity in your body with a good detox program. We will look at some unique studies where science proves the problems, and holistic therapies and healthy foods give us the chance to heal. We need to understand the problems, learn how to make the changes and how to make sensible choices for the healthiest baby possible. If your child already has a disease, this book is loaded with helpful information to make some positive health changes for you, your family and children.

232 Toxins in Baby Umbilical Cords

"What big eyes we have" to see the frightening studies in the next chapter, "Who's Afraid of the Big Bad Wolf." You will see how our children are starting life with an average of 27 toxins discovered in their umbilical cords. We need to "cut the cord" on Toxins!

Funny Fat Cartoons Characters

"Hey, Hey, Hey... Its Fat Albert" and Fred Flintstone and Homer Simpson and they are all here to make us laugh. However, back in the 60's and 70's, fat kids were scarce. It is no laughing matter that 1 out of every 3 kids are overweight today. We need to take discipline very seriously; the strength to discipline ourselves to help us stay strong and make the right food choices for our kids. Today's parents fall into a trap, the technology trap, meaning they want it now and they want it fast. Many parents turn to those fast processed foods for themselves and their kids. It is important to learn the science of food, especially carbohydrates and how our kids develop a love affair with them. When you add dairy, you have a match made in heaven like "mac & cheese." We need to remember that we are the teachers and our kids are the students. If you feed your kids carbs and dairy, your kids are going to be less interested in the healthy foods like vegetables and fruits. It is "better late than never" but the longer you wait, the tougher the battle on your war between healthy versus processed foods. When we come home tired, it is easy to cave when our kids refuse to eat, throw their food and cry when they do not get what they want. "May this source be with you!"

Mommy' Poppins

"So spit spot"...we should strive to be like Mary, practically perfect in every way. To do this we need to understand our own health and journey back to our childhood. Were we breastfed? Did we ingest antibiotics or were we pumped up with weekly allergy shots? Did we eat fast food, junk food, processed food, high quantities of white flour and sugar? A lifetime of toxins may be lurking inside your body; are our bodies ready for pregnancy?

"Chim Chim Cher-ee" ...We need more than good luck to get our bodies ready for pregnancy. When I see clients, including younger people, their number one complaint is they are tired and lacking energy. Many use coffee or energy drinks all day just to survive. This is not how we want to start our pregnancy. We need to make our engines strong and efficient. Our babies will be getting their nutrients, enzymes and vitamins from our body. If we start nutrient deficient and full of toxicity, our babies will not get what they need and you will be living off what little is left. So maybe we need to get our chimneys cleaned out, removing the soot of toxins and start to clean out our pipes.

Note: NO DETOXING IF YOU ARE PREGNANT. JUST GOOD HEALTHY FOODS AND SUPPORTIVE VITAMINS, MINERALS AND OILS. (See Chapter 23 on healthy hormone balance and supplements for pregnancy)

Smokey says "Stomp out your Campfires"

So let's put a fire in our belly and stomp out those toxins. I suggest reading my first book, *Why Can't I Lose Weight? Toxins.* This is a handbook that journeys through the stages of teaching you how to detox your body and to get rid of your toxic load. Not only did I heal from 18 diseases/disorders, I began sleeping through the night again; my hair grew in thicker and healthier than when I was a teenager and I look much younger at 58 than I did at 50. I was diagnosed with mostly autoimmune diseases: Hashimoto thyroid, fibromyalgia, type 2 diabetes, Adrenal Fatigue, Epstein Barr, IBS, Celiac mixed with other disorders like arrhythmia, vertigo and more. To add insult to injury I gained 50 pounds. My body was dying and I knew I was in trouble after a year of going to many medical doctors and showing no improvement. So, I took things into my own hands. I discovered that by healing naturally from my diseases, I could no longer pull the age card or the heredity blame. The real problem...toxicity and the real solution...detox!

Take a good look in the mirror! Do you look healthy or is there room for improvement? Our skin, hair and nails are an indication of how healthy or unhealthy we are on the inside. I had lost so much hair, had toenail fungus, dead root canal teeth and my skin looked old and wrinkled. These outer visual signs should be a wakeup call for everyone...they represent the increase of underlying diseases, inflammation and infections.

So cheer up "In every job that must be done there is an element of fun" so snap to the internet, pick up a copy of my previous book, *Why Can't I Lose Weight? Toxins* and let us have some fun getting rid of those toxins. It is not magical, you will have to do some work, but your reward is that you and your baby will live happily and healthily ever after.

If it looks like a duck...quacks like a duck...it must be a duck....Duh!!!

Let us Quack this case open! If we are born with toxins + eat toxins + drink toxins + scrub with toxins + breathe toxins + injected with toxins = we are full of toxins. Could this be the missing link to all children's and adult diseases including the 7 deadly diseases: Autism, ADHD, ADD, SIDS, Asthma, Diabetes and Obesity? Quack, Quack...

2

"WHO'S AFRAID OF THE BIG BAD WOLF" - TOXINS IN NEWBORNS

"Who's Afraid of the Big Bad Wolf?" I am. If you build your house with straw or twigs, then the big bad wolf will blow your house down. "Add another brick in the wall"; build your home strong so you will be able to protect your baby from the big bad toxins. When we are pregnant, we want to build our bodies with the strongest immune boosters of vitamins, minerals and enzymes, keeping both our immune systems strong.

"Here They Come to Save the Day" The Mighty EWG

We have a great organization and resource system that helps to keep us safe, the Environmental Working Group (EWG). They are a non-profit organization that enlists five laboratories in the U.S., Canada, and Europe. "The Environmental Working Group's (EWG) mission is to empower people to live healthier lives in a healthier environment. With breakthrough research and education, we drive consumer choice and civic action."

THE MOST SHOCKING PART OF THIS BOOK - PLEASE READ

In 2007 and 2008, the EWG organized laboratory testing of the umbilical cord blood of ten minority newborns. They confirmed nine out of the 10 tested positive for bisphenol, a (BPA) and 10 out of 10 tested positive for mercury and lead. BPA is a toxic plastic component, which is in the majority of plastics used today. **The lab identified 232 toxic industrial chemicals and pollutants in the umbilical cords from all ten babies.**

BPA is linked to many serious, chronic disorders including cancer, reproductive abnormalities, diabetes, asthma, obesity and cardiovascular abnormalities, etc. Mercury can cause nervous system disorders, respiratory failure, cancers and kidney damage.

Lead is harmful to nearly all systems of the body causing damage by harmful free radicals, especially in the brain.

There are limited amounts of studies conducted in the United States, but these two studies show evidence that American children are definitely exposed to toxins while in the womb and **toxins are crossing the placenta in large numbers to contaminate babies.**

Results from 336 Umbilical Cord Chinese Infants

- Reported pesticide exposure in cord blood for all 336 Chinese infants
- 75 of 96 pesticides/metabolites were detected in at least one sample
- 15 to 48 pesticides detected in their cord blood samples
- Infants born in the summer months had greater numbers of detected pesticides in their cord blood compared to infants born in the winter
- Levels for many of the pesticides measured in China, particularly pyrethroid insecticides, were higher than U.S. studies
- Prenatal pesticide exposure is a concern, because the fetal brain is rapidly developing in utero and pesticide exposure during this period of critical development may have long-lasting effects on neurodevelopment

This study was funded by R01ES021465 from the National Institute of Environmental Health Sciences (NIEHS), P01HD39386 from the National Institute of Child Health and Development (NICHD) and 81273085 from the National Natural Science Foundation of China (NNSFC).

http://www.ncbi.nlm.nih.gov/pmc/articles/PMC4730485/ (ENTIRE STUDY)

Infant Deaths in the United States 2013 - 2014

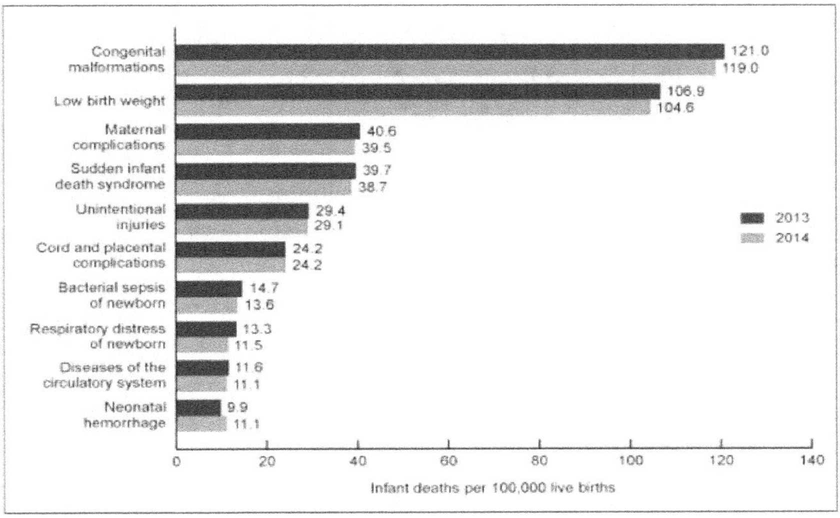

Many of the above causes of death can be linked to SIDS. Researchers have stated even though extensive research was conducted on SIDS, there are no known causes according to medical research. Since 1950, 70,000 new chemical compounds have been invented and released into our environment, yet very few of these chemicals were researched or tested to be safe for our children or ourselves. It sends a chill down my spine knowing how many dangerous chemicals are in every aspect of our children's lives today. Could this increase be responsible for the deaths of some of our children today?

Sudden Infant Death Syndrome (SIDS)

The NIH (National Institutes of Health) conducted a study to determine if common bacterial toxins are responsible or have a vaccine potential.

- Some of the evidence supports the hypothesis that common bacterial toxins are important in the causes of SIDS
- These bacterial toxins act as triggers to initiate a biochemical cascade resulting in death
- Data from research groups indicated that the bacteria Clostridium perfringens, Escherichia coli, **Staphylococcus aureus**, Streptococcus spp. and Enterococcus spp. **were present in higher numbers in infants who had suffered SIDS**

What SIDS and My Mercury Extraction have in Common

What I personally find interesting with this study are the common denominators of

- Mercury
- Illness for me/death for SIDS kids
- The infection, staphylococcus aureus

found between children dying from SIDS and myself who had 18 diseases in my body. **Staphylococcus aureus was found in children that died from SIDS and also found in the tissue that was tested from my extracted teeth.** I had 10 root canals and mercury filled teeth removed; all filled with infection. Below are the results showing the 15 infections found in just one of my extracted teeth. My assumption is babies who died from SIDS had mercury in their body from vaccines, where I had the same infection that came out of my 40-year-old mercury filled tooth. I carried a lifetime of infection and illness in my mouth until the last tooth extraction was complete. This shows how dangerous mercury can be to adults, let alone a tiny baby injected with chemicals, especially mercury.

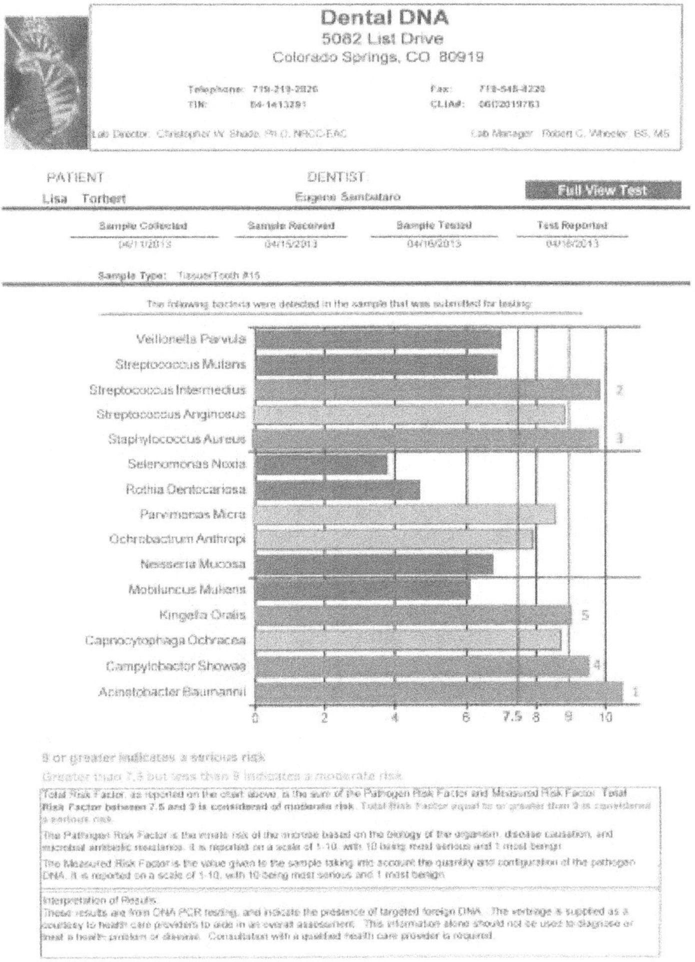

Dental DNA
5082 List Drive
Colorado Springs, CO 80919

PATIENT: Lisa Torbert
DENTIST: Eugene Santataro

Full View Test

Sample Collected	Sample Received	Sample Tested	Test Reported
04/11/2013	04/15/2013	04/16/2013	04/16/2013

Sample Type: Tissue/Tooth #15

Veillonella Parvula
Streptococcus Mutans
Streptococcus Intermedius 2
Streptococcus Anginosus
Staphylococcus Aureus 3
Selenomonas Noxia
Rothia Dentocariosa
Parvimonas Micra
Ochrobactrum Anthropi
Neisseria Mucosa
Mobiluncus Mulieris
Kingella Oralis 5
Capnocytophaga Ochracea
Campylobacter Showae 4
Acinetobacter Baumannii 1

0 2 4 6 7.5 8 9 10

9 or greater indicates a serious risk
Greater than 7.5 but less than 9 indicates a moderate risk

Total Risk Factor, as reported on the chart above, is the sum of the Pathogen Risk Factor and Measured Risk Factor. Total Risk Factor between 7.5 and 9 is considered of moderate risk. Total Risk Factor equal to or greater than 9 is considered a serious risk.

The Pathogen Risk Factor is the innate risk of the microbe based on the biology of the organism, disease causation, and microbial antibiotic resistance. It is reported on a scale of 1-10, with 10 being most serious and 1 most benign.

The Measured Risk Factor is the value given to the sample taking into account the quantity and configuration of the pathogen DNA. It is reported on a scale of 1-10, with 10 being most serious and 1 most benign.

Interpretation of Results
These results are from DNA PCR testing, and indicate the presence of targeted foreign DNA. The [illegible] is supplied as a courtesy to health care providers to aide in an overall assessment. This information alone should not be used to diagnose or treat a health problem or disease. Consultation with a qualified health care provider is required.

This is the lab test that was completed with the tissue extracted from just one of my root canal teeth. As you can see, I had 15 different infections from the one tooth. If you have root canals, they will hold infection until you have the teeth removed. A root canal kills the root and the tooth is now dead and capped off allowing infections to harbor for years. Read more in my book *Why Can't I Lose Weight? Toxins.*

3

"STRONG TO THE FINISH, CAUSE I EAT MY SPINACH" - WHAT TO EAT?

Popeye was a spinach pusher and when he ate his spinach, he would develop superhuman strength to clobber Bluto, when he ate his spinach. I'm not sure why he didn't push fish since he was a sailor man and his girlfriend's name was Olive Oyl. I can tell you that my brother and I both ate our spinach as young kids. This shows us how cartoon characters can highly influence our kids. We see how they relate to Ronald McDonald and Tony the Tiger too, asking for those unhealthy foods. Let's face it, cartoons can get our kids to eat better than we can.

Below are charts for healthy eating options where portions will vary depending on the age of your child, if you are pregnant or nursing or just for good healthy eating. The basis is a healthy protein, carbohydrate and fruit at every meal with unlimited veggies. I highly recommend eating organic meats and veggies, Non GMO, no dairy and wild caught seafood only. Make sure adults are eating at least 5-6 servings of non-starch vegetables a day. Make sure kids start eating vegetables early. If they do not like them, keep trying and alternate with different varieties. These are the super antioxidants of life and the most important food in their diet. The more raw foods as well as veggies and fruits ingested, the more vitamins, enzymes, and minerals your body will absorb.

What to Eat During Pregnancy and When Nursing

- 5 - 6 servings of vegetables
- 5 - 7 servings of carbohydrates
- 2 or 3 servings of fish a week
    - Fish lower in mercury: salmon, shrimp, pollock, tuna (light canned), catfish, and cod.
    - Avoid 4 types of fish: tilefish from the Gulf of Mexico, shark, swordfish, and king mackerel. Limit white (albacore) tuna to 6 ounces a week.
- No white rice due to arsenic (use brown, black & wild)
- Do not eat peanut butter (grown in the ground, very moldy)
- Do not eat grapes or raisins (highest pesticides, green organic are ok)
- No alcohol
- Stop smoking
- Eat at least 3 servings of organic protein only (limit beef, chicken, pork, or buffalo to once a week)
- Incorporate beans into your diet (they contain protein, carbs and are high in iron)

- Eat the following – Foods containing natural iron: mircrograms (mg)

Soybeans, cooked	1 cup	8.8 mg
Blackstrap molasses	2 tbsp	7.2 mg
Lentils, cooked	1 cup	6.6 mg
Spinach, cooked	1 cup	6.4 mg
Chickpeas, cooked	1 cup	4.7 mg
Tempeh	1 cup	4.5 mg
Lima beans, cooked	1 cup	4.5 mg
Black-eyed peas, cooked	1 cup	4.3 mg
Swiss chard, cooked	1 cup	4.0 mg
Kidney beans, cooked	1 cup	3.9 mg
Black beans, cooked	1 cup	3.6 mg
Pinto beans, cooked	1 cup	3.6 mg
Turnip greens, cooked	1 cup	3.2 mg

- Calcium Recommendations Instead of Dairy

Bok Choy	222 mg	3 cups
Collard greens	360 mg	3.5 cups
Kale	300 mg	3 cups
Tofu	434 mg	½ cup
Milk	305 mg	1 cup (**Not recommended**)
Broccoli	129 mg	3 cups
Sesame seeds	264 mg	3 tbsp

- No cheese (if you can't give it up, use only organic hard cheese aged 6 months or more)
- No nitrates (bacon, hot dogs, sausage, cold cuts)
- Make your own nitrate-free sausage with ground chicken. Slice your own organic meat for next day lunches.
- No processed fruit or vegetable juice (buy a juicer and make your own)
- Limit coffee to 8 oz., organic, not to exceed 16 oz. per day (none when nursing)
- No smoked meats
- Drink at least 8 cups of water a day (64 oz.)

Babies Newborn – 24 Months - Breast Milk Please

0 – 24 months - Breast Milk is the MOST IMPORTANT source of nutrition for your infant up to 12-24 months of age. Do NOT replace or introduce any solid foods into your baby's diet until your pediatrician gives you the go ahead. I highly recommend breast milk to any formula for your baby. I will go as far to say I would reconsider even having a child if you are not going to breast feed. **We have a fast food epidemic; we do not want to bring into the world, a fast food baby.** The odds will be stacked against your babies health early in life. It will take a little more time, but the investment will be well worth it. You will need to be organized and dedicate time to pumping for daycare.

Storing Breast Milk

Room temperature Freshly pumped breast milk can be kept at room temperature for up to four hours. If it is extremely hot in your home, reduce to 2 hours.

Insulated cooler Freshly pumped breast milk can be kept in an insulated cooler with ice packs for up to eight hours.

Refrigerator Freshly pumped breast milk should be stored in the back of the refrigerator for up to three days.

Freezer Freshly pumped breast milk can be stored in the freezer for up to 6 months. When removing milk from the freezer, use within 2 days. When thawing out, place milk in the refrigerator the night before or place it in warm water, never microwave.

If your child is sick or hospitalized, you will need to follow the guidelines set forth by your doctor. You will most likely be directed to use only fresh breast milk.

6-8 months Introducing Foods

The MOST IMPORTANT part about introducing foods to your baby is the 4 day plan. You will introduce only one food at a time for four days in a row to make sure your baby does not have an allergic reaction to it. Here are the foods to introduce first:

- 100% oatmeal or amaranth, not instant products (best choice)
- Cooked brown rice cereal, not instant (limit - READ ARSENIC IN RICE CHAPTER 14)

- Avocado – fresh (just mash up)
- Banana – fresh (just mash up)
- Organic peaches – fresh (just cut up)
- Organic soft fruit and when teeth develop, harder fruits cut up small such as apples and pears (use a bullet or blender and add harder fruit like apples then blend and serve. That's it…very easy and fresh)
- Organic veggies - beans, asparagus, kale, spinach, any veggie – (use bullet to puree and serve)
- Scrambled eggs with tested veggies. Try plain eggs during the 4 day test but limit eggs to 1x a week.

I recommend making your child's baby foods. It is so easy and fast; everyone has 60 seconds to devote and you will save a ton of money. I recommend NOT to buy any jarred baby food, canned food, processed boxed foods, etc. If you have to in a pinch, buy organic jarred food (no plastic) and new bagged fruits and veggies.

What to Feed your 8 – 15 month Kids

When you first offer finger foods to your 8 month old, you will need to be very careful about your choices. They will need to be dissolvable and small soft foods. Don't play games and start the feeding struggles, feeding is serious business. Feed them or let them feed themselves and make sure to join them at the dinner table. Pick soft and easily chewed foods that they can eat with a fork, spoon or their fingers. Let them do it their way, don't force the silverware. Give them a selection of protein, carbs, and fat; let them choose what they are going to eat and in what order. Once you establish healthy eating habits and behaviors at the table, your kids will be well behaved at a restaurant too. Kids love to push buttons, even at an early age. Please remember you are the adult and teacher, they are not in charge. Set routine times for all meals. Use the sensible meals and limit the amount of snacks so your child will be hungry at dinnertime. If they start to throw their plate or silverware, just take it away and say no. If they start to throw their food it is most likely because it's a food they do not like. Use an empty bowl and tell them to put it in the bowl. Tell them we do not throw our food away. Limit what you put on their plate and make sure they are hungry. Limit snacks so there is not an issue with eating at mealtimes.

When children can hold their own cup, start to put the breast milk in their cup. At this point you can start to reduce time on the breast.

12 months and older

Serve your healthy dinner to your child. It's as easy as that. They eat what you are eating. If still developing teeth, puree their food.

"You say YES....I say Yes"

1. Real Oatmeal, not prepacked, not instant, plain cooked oatmeal. You can make it in a crock pot or pan and make enough for three days. Serve with fruit & raw nuts
2. Banana sliced in half with almond, cashew or walnut butter in the middle makes a sandwich...roll in nuts...drizzle only a little raw honey over it
3. French Toast - No enriched or bleached breads. Best grains are Organic amaranth, brown rice, or quinoa grains. Use bananas on top or almond butter with a little raw honey
4. Toast - Best grains are Organic amaranth, brown rice, quinoa grains; toast and top with bananas and a nut butter
5. Make Muffins (Make a dozen and save in refrigerator or freezer) Apple, cinnamon and strawberry no junk muffins. There are many great muffin recipes on the internet.

    Muffins

    2 apples shredded

    3 eggs

    2/3 cup unsifted Organic amaranth, brown rice, quinoa, or teff, gluten-free

    2 tsp cinnamon

    1/4 cup 100% maple syrup or raw honey

    2 tbsp olive oil or coconut oil

1 cup mashed banana
1 cup pineapple

Directions:
Preheat oven to 350 degrees. Whisk the eggs with the maple syrup, cinnamon and olive oil (or gently melted coconut oil). Grate the apples and stir into the egg mixture with one cup banana. Then fold in the self-rising flour. If using grain flours you will need to add in baking powder. Spoon into greased muffin tins, and bake for approximately 20 minutes, until golden and cooked in the center. Stick a toothpick in the center to test if done.

6. Scrambled Eggs – scramble eggs (a dozen at at time and put in BPA free containers). Pull out every morning and serve with Organic amaranth, brown rice, quinoa, or teff bread
7. Bean burrito – use the above eggs. Add your beans of choice. Roll up in tortilla made with organic amarath, brown rice, quinoa or teff grains and wrap up in BPA free plastic wrap
8. Banana pancakes made with Organic amaranth, brown rice, quinoa or teff (make up a dozen and freeze them in BPA free plastic)
9. Toast with apple butter
10. Smoothie recipes (from Chapter 15)
11. Scrambled eggs or omelets with veggies (spinach, garlic, tomatoes, and colored peppers)

How do we get them to eat healthy?

We love our kids and deep down we really want them to be healthy. It is easier if we start out with healthy foods, but if not, now is the time to make a change. If they don't like something, give them something else and try the food again next week. If we feed our kids the addictive foods like white flour and cheese, they will not have an appetite for the healthy foods because they are already addicted. Your children will not just change automatically from a happy meal to a smoothie right away; expect a transition period.

My suggestion is to start to phase out or cut the bad foods in half and mix something healthy in with it. For example, if they like mac and cheese, you will cook up a portion of zucchini and mix it in with the carb; over time continue to reduce the amount of pasta, increasing the zucchini. You can even puree the zucchini and mix it in, then it is invisible. Cut and dry, you need to make cooked homemade healthy food...period! Tell your child that they may have more of any of their favorite foods once he or she eats just the small amount of the healthier ones. By keeping it small, your child is motivated to try new foods. Even the pickiest of eaters will eventually be willing to take one bite of a hated food to get to one he or she likes. There may be some tears, but what is more important? What they eat now will set the path for their dietary lifestyle as an adult!

When you first start to make healthier foods, your kids will test you. Don't cave! Don't be a pushover. You need to take baby steps. They may even refuse to eat, so stay calm and don't push them. It will take some time, but they will be eating healthy before you know it. If they ask for more of the unhealthy food, the mac and cheese, let them know they have to eat the beans first. Explain to them they have to eat the food they were given because this is what is being served. Don't bribe or beg them to eat. Tell them it is healthy, good for them and tastes good. Tell them they are expected to eat it!

Pack your Kid's Lunch with Love & Well-being

Pack your lunch and your kids' lunch. The school lunch is nothing but a mess of prepackaged processed junk. You will save money and your health. Here are a few quick ideas:

1. Gluten Free Mexican Mini Quiches

   Organic cooked chicken or beef shredded or a vegan alternative meat
   1/2 cup shredded organic dairy free cheese alternative shreds
   (4 ounce) can mild green chilies, diced
   1/2 cup gluten free all-purpose flour
   1/2 teaspoon baking powder

1/2 cup dairy free plain almond milk with 1 teaspoon lemon juice stirred into it
1/4 cup dairy free sour cream alternative
2 large organic eggs, lightly beaten
2 tablespoons fresh chives, minced (minced then measured)
1/4 cup cilantro leaves, minced plus more for serving
1 cup homemade salsa (put peppers, onions, garlic, lime juice, cilantro, dash pink salt and blend. Quick and delicious)

Directions:
Preheat oven to 375 degrees. Lightly spray a standard muffin pan with cooking spray. In a large mixing bowl combine all the ingredients with a spoon until well mixed. Spoon the mixture into the prepared muffin tins. Bake for 30 minutes or until brown and set. Run a dinner knife around the edges of the quiches, remove from the pan and serve with your favorite salsa, add some extra sour cream and cilantro.

2. Make a sandwich with 2 pieces of Organic amaranth, brown rice, farro, quinoa, or teff (cut off the crust to make it fun). Add almond or cashew butter and sliced bananas; add a little honey as a treat.
3. Egg salad sandwich. Make up and store for a couple days of use. Use vegenaise or oil only mayo. Make sure to buy organic free roaming chicken eggs.
4. BLT – imitation bacon, avocado, lettuce and tomatoes rolled up in a tortilla.
5. Tuna sandwich on gluten free bread.
6. Tuna wrap - mix tuna with avacado, celery and onion.
7. Wild cooked shrimp, oil mayonnaise, lemon juice, chopped celery and fresh tarragon and black pepper in a gluten free pita.
8. Bean Wrap - whisk 1 part lemon juice to 2 parts olive oil; season with black pepper. Add finely chopped shallots and garlic, then toss with rinsed cannellini beans (white kidney beans), avocado, thinly sliced cucumber half-moons, and chopped fresh dill

9. Quick stir fry – Scramble 4 eggs, put aside. Saute' thinly sliced scallions or onions in vegetable oil, then add frozen organic carrots, peas, corn combo and a splash of water with organic soy sauce. Cook until heated through, then stir in leftover brown rice and a splash of water if needed. Add eggs back in. Top with toasted sesame seeds, and chopped walnuts.
10. Scrambled egg sandwich – Stir fry chopped cremini (mushrooms) with light organic Bragg's liquid aminos. Place on top of a gluten free bagel. Top with tomato and scrambled egg.

"NO NO NO I Don't Eat it No More"

Eliminate ALL prepackaged cereals, frozen breakfast foods, cereal bars, frozen pancakes and waffles, etc. If they are low in sugar, they are higher in sodium and many still have corn syrup or other corn products, dyes, and GMO's.

Breakfast for Champions" and it's not Cereal

You have already seen here that 1 out of every 3 kids are overweight and many have diabetes. If you look at the list of cereal ingredients, you can start to get an idea as to why our kids are so unhealthy. Every one of these processed, high sugar, GMO cereals are just junk food, meaning there are no nutrients in them. They just set your child up for the next sugar fix at lunch, the after school snack, dinner, and dessert. So we have to cut the crap and that means all processed foods, fast foods, white bread sandwiches and yes, even pizza. **YOU HAVE TO SET ASIDE TIME TO PREPARE AND COOK HEALTHY MEALS.** If you cook ahead, your life can be so much easier and your child will grow up eating real food, not processed white flour and sugar; which you have now learned, white flour = white sugar. Our bodies will process both as sugar. Remember, if a cereal states it is low in sugar, it may be higher in sodium; and many contain corn syrup or other corn by-products, dyes, and may be genetically modified (GMO) product.

"Lions & Tigers & Bears...Oh My"

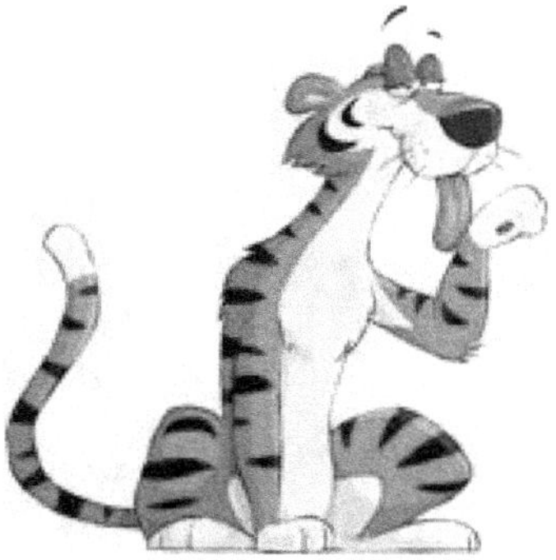

Bunnies, Bees, Toucans and Cuckoo birds are all playing a musical game on your children's heartstrings

Sugar content per one cup serving

Sugar - 10 grams "Brings out the tiger in you!" Frosted Flakes, **Your kids turns into crazy fighting Tigers**

Sugar - 9 grams "What are you eating? Nuttin' honey." **Yeah nuttin nutritious!**

Sugar - 14 grams "Can't get enough Super Sugar Crisp" & "Quisp for Quazy Energy" **Sugar Bear says "Sugar, Wheat, Corn Syrup, Honey, Caramel Color, and Salt... are my ingredients...crazy hyperactive energy!"**

Sugar - 9 grams "It's a honey of an O"... It's Honey Nut Cheerios. **Are you nuts? More sugar than honey plus cornstarch and brown sugar syrup.**

Sugar - 3 grams "Kid tested. Mother approved" Kix Cereal. **Maybe Kid approved and Mothers need to test it!**

Sugar - 9.4 grams "Honey-Comb's big! Yeah, Yeah, Yeah!" **Big on sugar, low on nutrition; over 2 tsp of sugar in every bowl.**

Sugar - 18 grams "Two scoops of raisins"...Kellogg's Raisin Bran **Two scoops of sugar 1 ½ cups per box and non-organic raisins equals dried pesticides in every bite.**

Sugar - 10 grams "A is for Apple, J is for Jacks." **A is for addictive. J is for Junk.**

Sugar - 4 grams "Snap! Crackle! Pop!" Rice Krispies **Snap, Crackle, Flop...robs you of energy.**

Sugar - 12 grams "Follow my nose. It always knows." Fruit Loops **It knows alright, something stinks here.**

Sugar - 10 grams "I'm cuckoo for Cocoa Puffs!" and **I'm cuckoo for buying this for my kids.**

Sugar - 10 grams "They're Magically Delicious!" Frosted Lucky Charms... **Let's make these disappear!**

Sugar - 10 grams "Silly Rabbit, Trix are for kids!" **Let's quit playing Trix on our kids...not nutritious.**

Sugar - 1 gram " Clinically Proven To Help Reduce Cholesterol" Cheerios **Because it has fiber….what a stretch. However, this is the winner for the lowest sugar and healthiest.**

A Lifetime Lifestyle for the Entire Family to Follow

Breakfast Ideas – Approximately 24 Grams Protein

Choose One Adult serving – Reduce for Kids

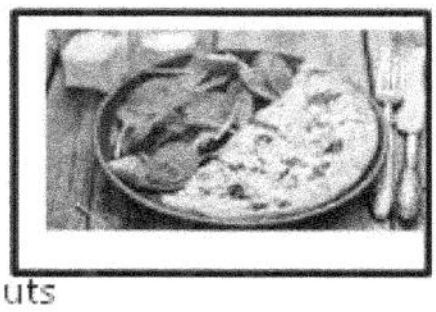

Eat It

- One large egg, veggies, brown rice, 1 serving of fruit
- Organic amaranth cereal or oatmeal with dates and walnuts
- Sweet potato mashed with one egg fried to a pancake, top with fruit
- Red potatoes, onions, black beans

Drink It

- 1 cup 25 calorie unsweetened nut milk (almond, cashew, coconut), 2-3 tbsp plant-based protein powder, 1 fruit, 1 tbsp nut butter (almond, cashew, coconut, walnut), 1 tbsp ground (hemp, chia or flax seeds) (organic pea protein, sweet potato protein)

Fruits and Serving Sizes – Three a Day

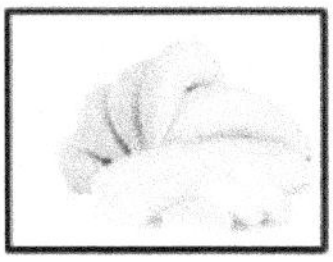

Bananas Chopped Fruit

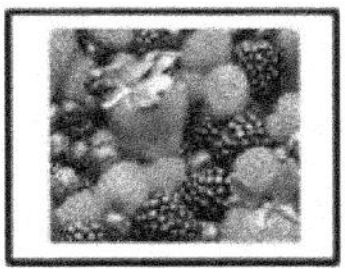

Hard Fruit

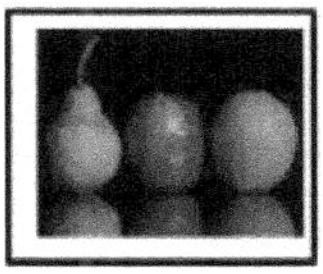

One Banana **½ Cup Chopped** **Size of a baseball**

Dirty, Buy Organic – Apples, grapes, strawberries, nectarines, peaches, blueberries, blackberries

Cleaner, can Buy Conventional – Bananas, pineapple, watermelon, canteloupe, grapefruit, mango papaya, kiwi, oranges

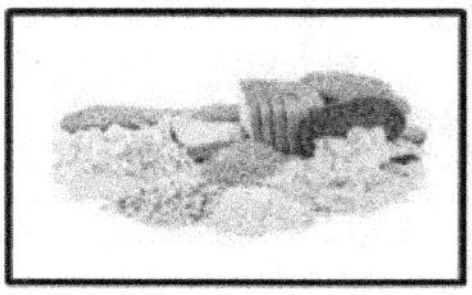

Complex Carbohydrates

Pick 1 for Breakfast, Lunch & Dinner Less for Kids

½ cup – Legumes, lentils, all beans, chickpeas, edamame

1 cup fresh or frozen starchy veggies – Parsnip, plantain, winter squash (acorn, butternut)

½ cup – carrots, green peas, pumpkin (No Corn)

1 cup or one medium – sweet potato or red potatoes (best)

½ cup –not enriched or bleached flour, Organic amaranth, oats, brown rice, brown rice pasta, farro pasta, quinoa, quinoa pasta, teff. Measure Oatmeal (dry), pasta (dry), quinoa (cooked), black, brown or wild rice (cooked), farro (dry), bread, pitas, wraps (low sugar)

Organic Protein - Approximately 20 grams

Pick 1 Breakfast, Lunch & Dinner –Less for Kids

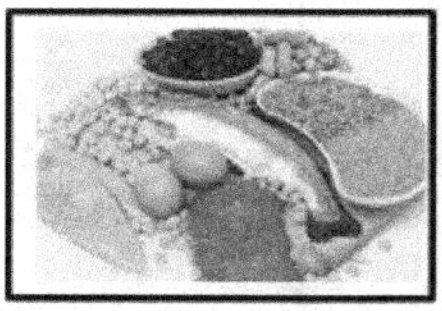

Eat 1 – 6 times per week
4 oz. –All fish Wild Caught and seafood ONLY,
(see chapter 17 for best choices)
5 oz. –Lobster (wild caught), Scallops (wild caught)
8 oz. – Crabmeat, clams (wild caught)
18 –Medium shrimp or oysters (wild caught)

Plant-Based **(unlimited)**: Organic pea protein, rice protein, sweet potato protein

3 oz. –Organic ground Chicken, lean red meat (beef, buffalo, lamb) (Must be grass fed, hormone/antibiotic-free) **Only 1 x per week**

4 oz. –All beans except baked beans and lima beans (starch), **unlimited**

2 eggs (organic) **limit 3 times per week**

Snacks – 3 fat servings a Day – Less Serving Size for Kids

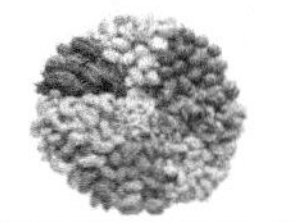

Organic Raw Nuts – 1 oz. Almonds (23), Brazil (7), Hazelnuts (20), Pine (160), Macadamia (11), Pecans halves (19), Walnuts halves (14), Pistachios (49), Cashews (18) NO PEANUTS

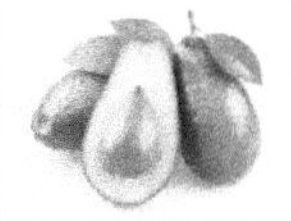

Avocado – ¼ of an avocado

Nut Butters – 2 tbsp. Almond, Cashew, Walnut, Seed Butters (raw best or r lightly roasted, organic), pink sea salt only

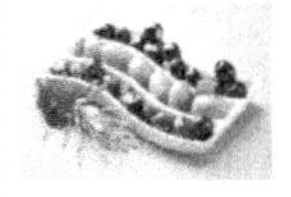

Olives – 10 jumbo olives (green or black)

Seeds – ¼ cup of sunflower or pumpkin seeds

Oils – Organic Walnut oil, Olive oil, Sesame oil, Flax oil, Coconut oil – 1 tbsp.

Best Sweeteners

- Organic maple syrup (grade B only– which does not contain formaldehyde)
- Organic date sugar
- Raw, unpasteurized honey
- Organic molasses
- Stevia

(No agave syrup, artificial sweeteners, corn syrups, cane sugar, brown sugar, brown rice sugar) These are processed and GMO products.

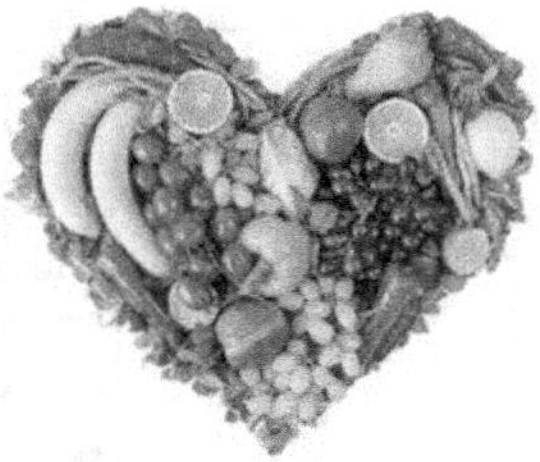

Unlimited Non-Starchy Vegetables

The Antioxidants of our Life

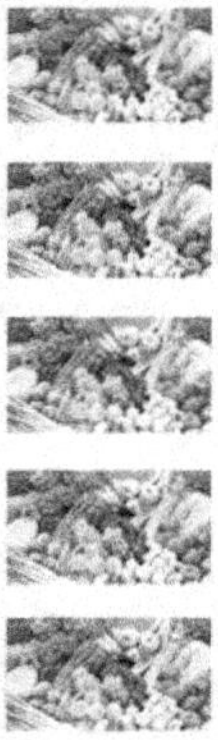

Artichokes
Asparagus
Bamboo Shoots
Beets
Bok Choy
Brussel Sprouts
Okra
Onions
Pea pods
Peppers
Radishes
Broccoli
Cabbage
Cauliflower
Cucumber
Daikon
Eggplant
Rutabaga
Spaghetti Squash
Sprouts
Sugar snap peas
Swiss chard
Fennel
Garlic
Green Beans
Jicama
Leeks
Mushrooms
Tomato
Turnips
Water Chestnuts
Wax beans
Zucchini

Greens (collard, kale, mustard, turnip, chicory, endive, escarole, lettuce, romaine, spinach)

AVOID THESE HIGHLY PESTICIDE FOODS

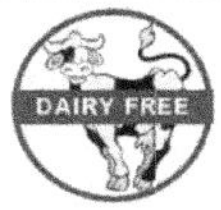

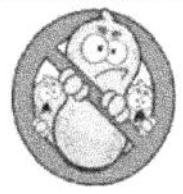

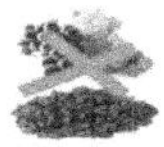

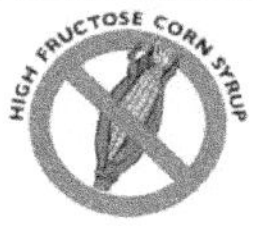

NO PEANUT OR PEANUT BUTTER – Moldy, grown in the ground, heavypesticides

Alternatives: Almond, Cashew, Walnut, and Seed and Butters

NO GRAPES OR RAISINS – Very heavy pesticides, grapes dried = raisinspesticides locked inside (**Organic green grapes OK**)

Best Alternatives: Try organic mango, papaya, dates, cranberries that are organic with no sugar added.

NO DAIRY – No cheese, yogurt, milk, butter or products that contain milk

Best Alternatives: Nut milks, cheese alternatives, nut cheeses, nutritional yeast

NO CORN – No GMO corn, cornmeal, corn syrup, corn starch, polenta, cornflour, popcorn. Corn is in almost every processed food, soda, salad dressing

NO SOY – No Soy, soy sauce, edamame, miso, soy protein, tofu, tamari, tempeh, textured vegetable protein, soybeans, Soya, Shoyu

NO OR LIMITED WHEAT – gluten, high-gluten flour, high-protein flour, vital gluten, wheat gluten, wheat starch, enriched flour, wheat germ, flour, starch, farina, modified starch, bran, vegetable starch, wheat bran, gelatinized starch, vegetable gum, graham flour, semolina, durum, couscous, cracker crumbs, einkorn, emmer, farina, farro, kamut, seitan, fu, spelt, sprouted wheat, triticale

Best Alternatives - Farro wheat, an ancient grain, Organic amaranth, brown rice, brown rice pasta, farro pasta, quinoa, quinoa pasta, teff

These are recommendations from the Environmental Working Group (EWG) for purchasing organic or conventional. If you buy conventional, clean well and cut off the skin. Organic will also need to be cleaned well.

EWG's Dirty Dozen + Two - Buy These Organic

1. Strawberries
2. Apples
3. Nectarines
4. Peaches
5. Celery
6. Grapes
7. Cherries
8. Spinach
9. Tomatoes
10. Sweet bell peppers
11. Cherry tomatoes
12. Cucumbers

+ Hot Peppers
+ Kale / Collard greens

EWG Clean Fifteen List - Buy Conventional

1. Avocado
2. Sweet Corn
3. Pineapples
4. Cabbage
5. Sweet peas frozen
6. Onions
7. Asparagus
8. Mangos
9. Papayas
10. Kiwi
11. Eggplant
12. Honeydew Melon
13. Grapefruit
14. Cantaloupe
15. Cauliflower

4

"MONSTERS INC." ADHD, AUTISM, & ALL KIDS

What Every Child Needs to Follow To Be Healthy

This chapter has good healthy choices for kids with ADHD, ADD, Autism and all kids to prevent illness, boost the immune system, help them heal and become healthy. There is a separate chapter for Autism, which will go into more specifics, especially with behavior.

According to the US Center for Disease Control, the national rate of Attention-Deficit/Hyperactivity Disorder (ADHD) is **(6.4 million) diagnosed with ADHD.**

- Approximately 11% of children 4-17 years of age (6.4 million) are diagnosed with ADHD as of 2011.
- The percentage of children with an ADHD diagnosis continues to increase, from 7.8% in 2003 to 9.5% in 2007 and to 11.0% in 2011.
- **Boys (13.2%) were three times more likely than girls (5.6%) to have ever been diagnosed with ADHD.**
- Males are almost three times more likely to be diagnosed with ADHD than females.
- During their lifetimes, 12.9 percent of men will be diagnosed with the attention disorder. Just 4.9 percent of women will be diagnosed.
- The average age of ADHD diagnosis is 7 years old.
- Symptoms of ADHD typically first appear between the ages of 3 and 6.

ADHD isn't just a childhood disorder. Today, about 4 percent of American adults over the age of 18 deal with ADHD on a daily basis.

See more: http://www.healthline.com/health/adhd/facts-statistics-infographic#1

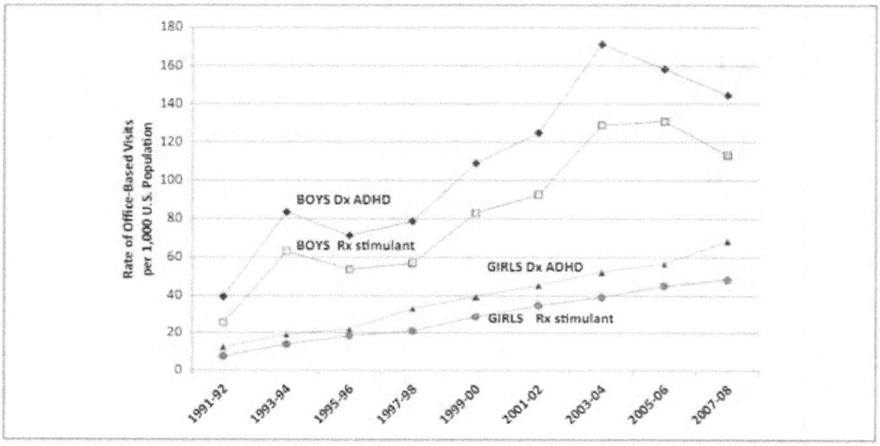

Figure 1. Annualized rate of office-based visits per 1000 US population aged 5 through 18 years with a diagnosis (D_x) of attention-deficit/hyperactivity disorder (ADHD), and rate with a D_x of ADHD and use of (R_x) a stimulation or atomoxetine, by gender

Attention Deficit-Hyperactivity Disorder (ADHD) is one of the most controversial issues parents have to deal with concerning the well-being of their children. I would like to discuss symptoms to look for, medication and natural alternative approaches to this disorder.

ADHD, as described in the Diagnostic and Statistical Manual of Mental Disorders (DSM IV), "is a persistent pattern of inattention and/or hyperactivity-impulsivity that is more frequent and severe than is typically observed in individuals at a comparable level of development." It affects mostly school-age kids, targeting more males than females. Teenagers as well as adults are also affected with ADHD. It usually is present before age seven. Many symptoms are seen at home and in school. The neurological conditions present three primary symptoms: a decreased ability to pay attention and focus on activities, difficulty controlling one's impulses and increased motor activity.

The following is a list of behaviors that may appear in ADHD children most of the time:

1. Fidgets and squirms
2. Difficulty remaining seated in school and at home
3. Is easily distracted
4. Has difficulty waiting their turn in games
5. Interrupts frequently
6. Has trouble following instructions
7. Has difficulty sustaining attention
8. Shifts from one activity to another
9. Talks excessively
10. Does not listen to what is said
11. Often loses things
12. Engages in dangerous activities
13. Often acts impulsively
14. Is often accused of over-reacting
15. Often feels life is overly stressful

Although many children possess some of these common behaviors, the difference when identifying ADHD is the repetition and frequency of the symptoms listed above. A child with ADHD may have many of the symptoms, year after year, at home, school and in day care. Often the child's behavior causes a negative reaction from parents, teachers and friends, causing the child's self-esteem to suffer. This increases the child's frustrations and keeps them locked in a downward spiral of destructive behavior.

Diagnosis is very controversial and requires medical professionals to spend a significant amount of time obtaining a detailed history from the parents. Direct observation in a familiar setting, such as school and home, are recommended to study the child's behavior. There are many reasons for children to have poor impulse control and attention including learning disabilities, hearing or visual impairment, behavior or psychiatric disorder and poor diet. Because the diagnosis is often unclear and complicated, it requires the consistent cooperation between the parents, teachers, psychiatrist, pediatrician and professional trained in testing for learning disabilities.

ADD/ADHD Kids Are Very Gifted Yet so Misunderstood

Many parents feel their kids have turned in to the abominable snowman and question who their kids really are. There is a lot of controversy, negativity, misdiagnoses and misunderstood children, which create even more stress on ADHD children and their parents. ADD/ADHD children need to find their niche by discovering their talents whether intellectual or sports related so they can believe how gifted they are. They need to feel included, not different or treated as outsiders. Besides being very gifted, ADHD people are the movers and the shakers of the world, including me!

Very Famous and Gifted ADHD/ADD People:

Inventors: Alexander Graham Bell, Thomas Edison, Albert Einstein, Benjamin Franklin

Entrepreneurs: Walt Disney, Bill Gates

Composers: Wolfgang Amadeus Mozart, Ludwig van Beethoven.

Presidents: Dwight D. Eisenhower, John F. Kennedy, Winston Churchill, Woodrow Wilson

Athletes: Terry Bradshaw, Michael Phelps, Cammi Granato, Michael Jordan, Babe Ruth

Actors: Jim Carrey, Ryan Gosling, Will Smith, Whoopi Goldberg, Suzanne Somers

Musicians: Justin Timberlake, Will.i.am, Ozzy Osbourne, Kurt Cobain, Steven Tyler, Elvis Presley, Stevie Wonder, Hayley Williams, Shakira, Hilary Duff, Zooey Deschanel, Cher Bono

Gifted Children

Something parents should consider is that if their children are gifted, they may be bored in school and exhibits lots of negative behavior and receive low grades as a result. Many gifted children do not pay attention, cause mischief, argue with teachers and have peer problems. It is easy to see why many of these children are linked in the diagnosis of ADH). A child can be gifted even if their IQ score is less than 130 since their creativity score is high. Gifted children often daydream and pay little attention in school because they are just not interested. Many of the school subjects seem boring and irrelevant to them. They also may challenge rules and engage in power struggles.

Gifted children are very emotional and passionate about their gifts. This list may include **music**, **singing**, **art, writing, drama, dance, and sports**. It is imperative to support their talents. Try to reason with them and reward them with weekend trips to concerts or sporting events, dancing, and arts and craft projects for doing well, or at least getting through the school week.

Musicians and singers develop very early, many times before they are a year old. If you notice they like to beat on a drum, make sure to have a little drum or some pots and pans handy. In addition, the little keyboards are nice where they introduce kids to beginner songs that only require a few keys. Kids will need adequate time to practice their instruments without interruption. It is necessary that you honor whatever type of music they enjoy from classical to jazz, blues, rock, metal, alternative, rap, hip-hop, country, etc. Maybe on the weekends they could learn a few of their favorites from a teacher at a music store. Let them pick their passion, a style they resonate with. They may enjoy playing different instruments.... let them! I play guitar, keyboard, percussion and I am a singer/songwriter, ADHD all the way! Some schools follow the mainstream of classical music and some are more creative with their choices. Another alternative is to find an after school groups that appeals to your child's interest. Here is an example of where a school used a popular song to show diversity: Pink Floyds "Dark Side of the Moon" Watch here:

https://www.youtube.com/watch?v=KhDKWdEhbkI.

Artists Most children love crafts. I can remember my mom telling me that I could not sit in front of the television without coloring. For those with ADHD, our brains process things differently. We find it easy to do more than one thing at once. We get bored easily. You may notice early on that your child loves to color and spends large amounts of their time invested in it. Using crayons, paint and colored pencils and different types of paper to change it up a bit. There are so many fun options with arts and crafts such as going to a pottery-craft business, working with sand, or perhaps a paint night where your child can paint with others. Weekend trips could include visiting an art museum or a craft fair.

Authors Writing is another great talent that your child may develop early on. You may notice they have a fascination with books at an early age. Their pens start to push on the paper creating poetry. Make sure to honor the poetry no matter how small. You could have fun with some rhyming words to help create some ideas for their writing. Weekend trips could include libraries, especially where they have scheduled authors or book readings or café bookstores where they can browse, read, and sip on some tea.

Drama and acting may start early, even as acting out. Of course, we are not acknowledging the latter. Here is where you can turn a negative into a positive, teaching them how to act out a book. Start with their favorite book and have them read the part of their favorite character where you read the other. The next step is starting to breathe some life into the characters, even dress the part. Weekend trips could include going to local plays to encourage their passion for acting/drama.

Dancing like a star starts very early in life, sometimes even before they can walk. I noticed my grandson loved to move his body to the beat when music came on. This can be a great reward by cranking up the volume and letting your child go. Kids love when you join in and give them a twirl or two. Later enroll them in ballet, tap, or a modern dance class where they can find their groove. Purchase age appropriate dance movies such as *Bring It On*, *Mad Hot Ballroom*, *Center Stage*, *Shall We Dance*, *Saturday Night Fever*, *Grease*, *Footloose*, *Flashdance*, and *Save the Last Dance*. Weekend trips to a ballet or dance show will be most enjoyable.

Sports This can be your best friend with an ADHD child. As you know, they have plenty of energy and are ready to unleash it. Some sports will require more coordination, so it is important to find a sport that your child really likes. Like anything else, the sport will always be more fun to them if they are good at it, not forcing them to play baseball because you are good at it. Make sure to go out and practice with your child, as they are not going to be a pro overnight. Weekend trips can be fun going to pro or statewide games in your hometown. See the breakdown on how to pick the right sport for your child later in this chapter.

If your gifted child continues to flounder in school, then maybe a more suitable solution would be to **change the school** (a private school or home-school) **instead of changing the child.**

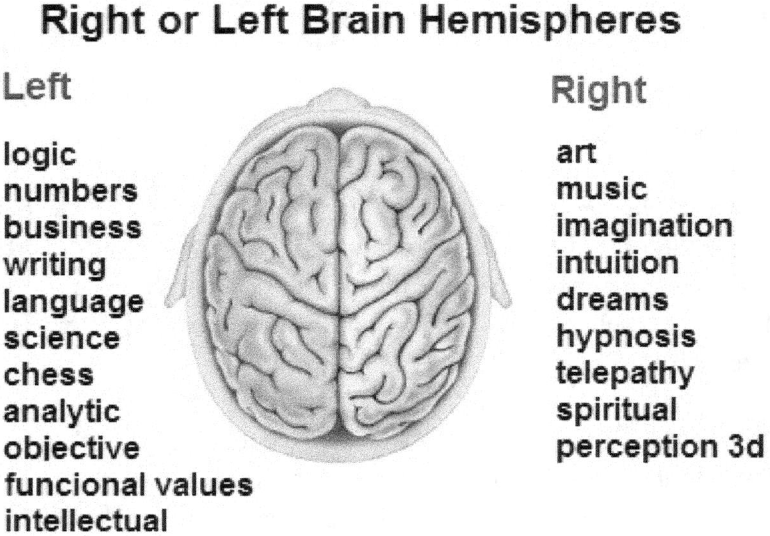

It helps to look at the above chart and see if your kids are more right or left brained thinkers. It is best to be able to understand these strengths and work with them instead of against them. Some will score more on the left side and others more on the right and some will be both or a combination of the two. There is a book entitled *Right-Brained Children in a Left-Brained World*. This is a great investment for right brained children, especially ones with ADHD. This book describes how visual thinkers learn differently and gives practical tips to incorporate into their education.

"See No Evil, Hear No Evil, Do No Evil" – How Your Child Learns

There are three different ways we learn, by seeing (visual), hearing (auditory), or doing (tactile-kinesthetic). Kids may learn from one or more of these learning styles. This is why it is so important to understand your child, to try different activities to see what your child likes and where their talents lie. When it comes to learning, it is essential to find out the best way your child learns. This can be important when working with a teacher and at home with you. Let us follow an example to show the three different ways to learn.

Putting the Puzzle Pieces Together

A. Teacher says this puzzle piece will be put in the top right (hearing)
B. Teacher shows you that the piece goes in the top right (seeing)
C. The child puts the piece in the top right (doing)

Visual Learners

Visual learners love to leaf through books and follow better when things are written on a blackboard or by following a graph. They need to see the information to process it, understand it and remember it. However, there are two types of visual learners. Picture learners will learn and explain or answer questions with pictures and graphs. Print learners think with words, are good at reading, spelling and writing, and learn to answer with just words.

Visual Learners Usually Have Some of the Following:

- Have trouble with following verbal directions
- Easily distracted by noise
- Like to read
- Good at spelling
- Memorize things by seeing them on paper
- Organized
- Would rather watch, than talk or do.
- Good handwriting
- Notice details
- Remember faces better than names
- Doodle on paper

Strategies That Help Visual Learners to Practice Reading

- Putting each letter on a card and have students arrange words
- Putting words on cards and have students arrange into sentences
- Putting sentences on paper strips to teach sequencing and paragraphing

Strategies That Help Visual Learners Practice Other Subjects

- Use visuals to teach lessons, including pictures, graphics, images, charts, outlines, story maps, and diagrams
- When giving verbal directions, write down key words or phrases and use visuals
- Demonstrate what you want your child to do
- Use dry erase boards with colored markers
- Use color cues, framing and symbols to highlight key information
- Encourage your child to write down and highlight key information
- Encourage the use of flashcards when memorizing (numbers, alphabet)
- Provide visual activities, including maps, videos, models, puzzles, matching activities, computers, and word searches

Advantages for Visual Learners

- They have a photographic memory – remember things with pictures
- Visionaries of the world – envision their future, big imagination and ideas
- Daydreamers – life is an adventure, are easily bored, think outside the box
- Artists, musicians - very creative
- Love using pictures – graphic artists
- Positive outlook - see beauty in all things
- Mind is constantly inventing and creating things
- Creative dresser (combining clothes), Interior decorator – arranging furniture

Strategies for Treating Hyperactivity - Dr. Oz & Dr. Fotuhi Brain Boosters

Dr. Oz Brain Booster #1: DHA

Essential fatty acid omega-3, called DHA, increases blood flow, decreases inflammation, reduces plaques in the brain. Take a good quality DHA daily to build memory and support the brain.

Dr. Oz Brain Booster #2: Brain Stimulating Switch-Ups

Use it or lose it; we need to exercise our brain muscles to build brain power:

- Put your watch on the opposite wrist
- Use opposite hand to brush your teeth and fix your hair
- Use other hand to eat
- Write backwards
- Dance

Dr. Oz Brain Booster #3: 7-7-7 Stress-Busting Breathing

Stress is poison to the brain, specifically the memory part; the hippocampus. People with high levels of anxiety, stress, experience apnea, snoring, are overweight, suffer from diabetes or hypertension and have high levels of cortisol, all of which can wreak havoc on the memory. The size of the brain can shrink 20-30% due to the effects of stress. Practice deep breathing to calm the nerves. Breathe in for a count of 7, hold for a count of 7, then exhale for a count of 7.

Dr. Oz Brain Booster #4: Tease Your Memory

We need to do activities that stretch brain abilities. Make an association game to help with memory. Start with four items on a grocery list: milk, eggs, hamburger, and an apple; make an association between them. Think of filling an egg with milk then smash the egg with an apple creating a mess that is wiped up with the hamburger meat.

Dr. Oz Brain Booster #5: Brain Push-Ups

Increasing your physical stamina and strength increases growth factors and can actually generate new brain cells. Building brain cells does not require operations or taking drugs, it is as simple as remembering lists, telling stories, and writing backwards. Dr. Fotuhi states "by doing seven or more push-ups a day, you can improve blood flow to the brain to support brain function and memory."

Dr. Oz Brain Booster # 6: Superfood to Save Memory

Big belly and weight gain cause the brain to shrink. Try any of these brain superfoods:

1. Elderberries – fresh, dried or juice. Energy for mitochondria
2. Pecans – choline. High in EFA (highest antioxidant nut)
3. Clams – B12, iron & zinc
4. Homemade vegetable juice. Gold mine for all known vitamins
5. Beets, radishes or cabbage. Natural nitrates to enhance blood flow to brain.

Are Your Road Runners Turning Taz – Kids Behavior

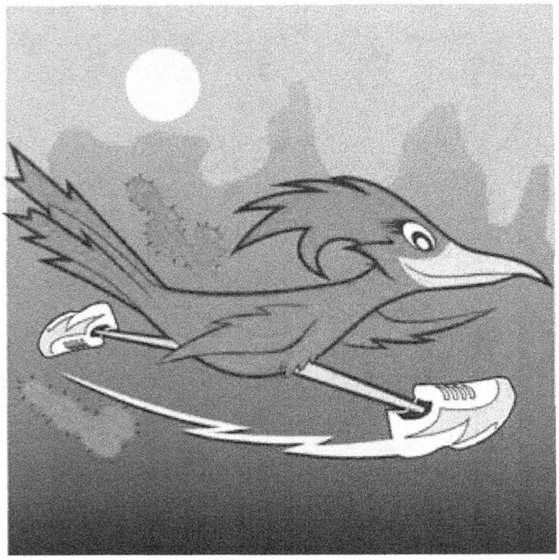

Some of our kids may be able to identify with Road Runner because they are always going 100 miles per hour. Others will be able to identify with the Looney Tunes Taz. He has no problem expressing his anger especially when he is whirling around like a cyclone. Sometimes his speech is peppered with growls, grunts, and fragmented sentences. He is going so fast he has trouble putting words together. Every child's temperament and behavior will have to be factored into the equation.

"If you're on the highway and Road Runner goes "Beep Beep",
Just step aside or you might end up in a heap.
Road Runner, Road Runner runs down the road all day.
Even the Coyote can't make him change his ways.

Road Runner, the Coyote's after you.
Road Runner, if he catches you you're through.
That Coyote's really a crazy clown!
When will he learn he never can mow him down?
Poor little Road Runner never bothers anyone;
Just runnin' down the road's his idea of having fun."

You will need to see if there is a temperament clash between your child and you, your spouse or a teacher. A quiet and reserved adult is more likely to be upset and see a problem with a child of an opposite temperament such as a high-energy extraverted child. In this type of situation, a child may receive vibes that the adults do not like him or her, which in turn produces anxiety, depression and acting out behaviors. It is important to understand what type of temperament your child has and to learn ways to deal with their behaviors. *Nurture by Nature* is a book, which helps people to understand how a child's mind works and how to interact with them.

Behavior modification techniques are often a positive reinforcement to change undesirable behavior. Using behavior modification techniques are an attempt to actually change the negative behaviors and teach the child more positive ways to interact. Parents have reported that "time outs" and rewarding with "smiley" faces work better than screaming and yelling at their children. It is very important to designate a specific amount of time each day for giving a child some positive attention. It seems like a simple task but can prove to be very difficult in the stressful lives we live.

Education is perhaps the best approach to this highly misdiagnosed disorder. The education I am talking about is for the parents, teachers and even the doctors. The natural approaches are certainly going to require parents and teachers to invest time every day with the child. Are you looking for a quick fix, an easy solution by tranquilizing your little roadrunner or a permanent solution? We really don't want to smash the life out of our crazy little clowns!

Twilight Zone – Medications

In our fast-paced world, many parents, teachers and doctors swear by medication as a solution to taming the wild beast. It is true that **medication can turn a spirited hyperactive child into a quiet compliant one. Many parents will have to decide for themselves: is this my goal?** Stimulant medications such as Ritalin, Dexedrine and Cylert can help normalize a child's behavior by producing a sedative effect. One of the most prescribed medications is Ritalin. Taking medications as treatment for ADHD is introducing drugs to your child at a very early age. The only difference between this and the street drug "Speed", is that the street drug is illegal. A drug is a drug is a drug, and they are very addicting. The other concern is that medications are only treating the symptoms, not the problem.

Children taking Ritalin have reported having adverse reactions including nausea, dizziness, heart palpitations, headaches, drowsiness, tachycardia, abdominal pain and weight loss. Many critics argue that medication is over prescribed and there are many other alternatives to research before medicating your children. The chart below shows 2,302,049 reported adverse reactions to the drugs. I will hope that these staggering statistics will deter the masses from introducing dangerous drugs to our young children.

The National Attention Deficit Disorder Association states that Methylphenidate (Ritalin) is a medically prescribed stimulant medication that does not cause addiction or dependence and does not lead to psychosis. However, below is a chart showing misuse or abuse of pharmaceuticals along with illicit drug use. As you can see the combination of these two is over 2 ½ million children and the misuse of pharmaceutical drugs is even higher than the illicit drugs.

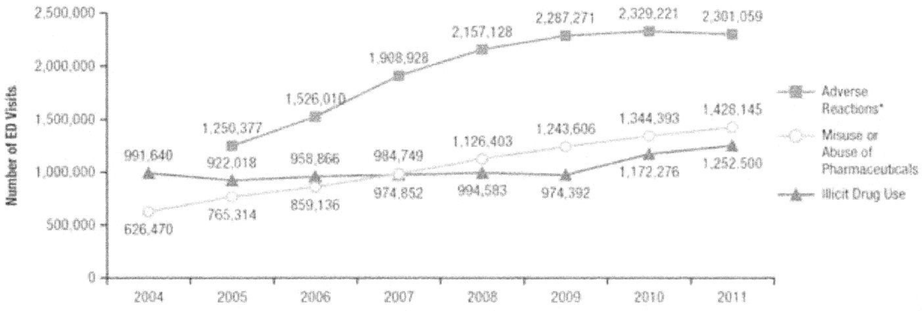

* The estimate for ED visits involving adverse reactions in 2004 was suppressed due to low statistical precision.
Source: 2011 SAMHSA Drug Abuse Warning Network (DAWN).

ADD/ADHD Medication

Ritalin and Adderall are medications used to treat conditions like Attention Deficit Disorder (ADD) and Attention Deficit Hyperactivity Disorder (ADHD). These are amphetamines and their main purpose is to speed up the body making it easier to focus. These drugs are highly addictive and cause side effects such as anxiety, hostility, exhaustion, and trouble sleeping. Many doctors will then give children a sleeping pill to help with insomnia. It breaks my heart that doctors that we trust would start young children on these drugs, setting them up for such an unhealthy life and possible addiction. These medications are very over prescribed.

Nutritional Supplements Work Equally Well for ADHD According to Study Results

Many parents decide to take the easy way out, using meds for their ADD/ADHD child, fearing poor academic performance during the school year. Most doctors seem to ignore government studies showing how supplements help with ADHD but instead, recommend medications supporting the pharmaceutical companies. There are compelling studies that show how brain chemistry imbalances from nutritional deficiencies are reversible by adding amino acids, vitamins, and mineral supplementation.

According to the NIH, "Although the use of natural medications for ADHD has been considered as a "safer" approach, natural products are still far from being called as standard ADHD treatments due to the lack of comprehensive and appropriately controlled clinical studies that interrogate both their efficacy and safety. Moreover, it is challenging to compare efficacy profiles of herb therapy with conventional pharmacological ADHD treatments, mainly because herbal preparations are not standardized, and question regarding their purity, reliability, safety, and toxicity profiles will always arise."

This study did show improvement for each of the following supplements and Amino Acids, using only one supplement in each study, not a combination of all supplements.

Supplements

1. Ginkgo Biloba
2. Bacopa
3. Ginseng Korean Red
4. Passion Flower
5. Pycnogenol
6. Zinc
7. EFA
8. Iron
9. Valerian
10. Yizhi

Amino Acids

1. Acetyl – L carnitine
2. Taurine
3. Glycine
4. L-theanine
5. L-tyrosine

For more information, read this study in its entirety. http://www.ncbi.nlm.nih.gov/pmc/articles/PMC4757677/

Brain Starvation

In the 1990's, Dr. Charles Gant, MD, PhD, NMD became best known for his work in biomolecular/nutritional medicine as it relates to brain physiology and psychotherapy. Due to the evidence of his study and others, he found that certain causative "risk factors" for ADHD clustered around eight areas:

- food allergies
- thyroid disorders
- amino acid deficiencies
- essential-fatty-acid deficiencies
- mineral deficiencies
- heavy metal toxicities
- B vitamin deficiencies
- High-carbohydrate-low protein diet

In simple terms, Dr. Gant suggests that scientific data strongly suggests that ADHD children (and adults) suffer from various combinations of brain starvation (mineral - vitamin deficiencies), brain poisoning (lead and toxic metals) or metabolic abnormalities (thyroid disorders), all of which can be discovered by simple laboratory tests of the blood, hair and/or stool.

Dr. Gant comments, "When a child's brain is poisoned with lead, reacting to food allergies or starving for essential fats, protein or zinc, why cover up symptoms with an amphetamine drug? The child's brain needs to have the lead removed, the food allergies neutralized and the deficiencies for essential fatty acids, protein and zinc replenished so that the symptoms can be resolved at their roots." Dr. Gant summarizes his two decades of clinical practice applying this approach in his book *ADD and ADHD: Complementary Medicine Solutions* (self-published) and *End Your Addiction Now* (Warner Books).

Nutritional supplementation consisted of a **multiple vitamin, a multiple mineral, phytonutrients, essential fatty acids (fish oil), phospholipids (soy lecithin), probiotics (acidophilus), detoxifying supplements and amino acids.** Both groups showed statistically valid and similar improvements, but the nutritionally supplemented treatment group did not suffer the side effects commonly experienced by children treated with Ritalin and other stimulant medication.

"One pill makes you higher and one pill makes you chill"

The ups and downs of daily medication can take its toll on a young body. It artificially speeds up the body, putting stress on all of the organs. The following are natural treatments that are worth the time to help re-evaluate the foods your family eats and to make the necessary changes.

"Cloud 9" – Nine Ways to Heal the Natural Way

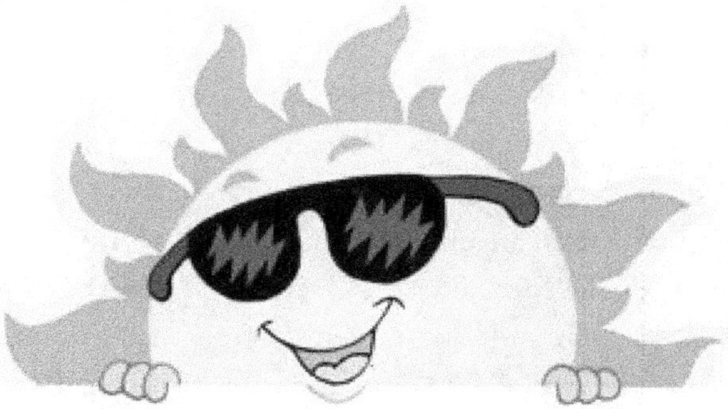

1. Drink plenty of water
2. Use pink sea salt
3. Get at least 5 consecutive hours of sleep
4. Exercise
5. No white flour, sugar - gluten free
6. Remove MSG & Food Dyes
7. Eat sulfur based foods
8. Play out in the Sun
9. Remove trans fats, use EFA, DHA and supplements

"Singing in the Rain" - Water

Since our brains are 85% water, they depend on a sufficient amount of water to function well. It is important to drink at least half your body weight in ounces of water a day. Example: Weight 70 pounds = 35 ounces of water. Water helps to hydrate the entire body and brain; all of our organs need water to survive. This means plain water, not soda, teas or anything with chemicals or sugar. Water also aids in the production of our feel good neurotransmitters, dopamine and norepinephrine. Grab a nice BPA free kid friendly container and fill it with good quality water, to help keep your child's brain focused.

"When It Rains, It Pours" – Pink Salt

It is important to add pink sea salt into your diet and your child's diet, excluding babies under 18 months old. Most of you have been told that salt is not good for you. You may have been told that it causes fluid retention. Iodized salt or table salt is not good for the human body because it is heated above

1,200 degrees, changing its chemical structure, which means you are ingesting a chemical toxin. This cheap salt can also contain aluminum and anti-caking agents, making it easier to pour. So toss the iodized salt or save it to put down on your walkways when it snows. Iodized salt is acid forming to the body, whereas sea salt produces an alkalizing effect. Iodine is important for hormone health. Since there is only a small amount of iodine in sea salts, alternatives will include eating seaweed, cod, shrimp and eggs. Premier Pink Salt, from Premier Research Labs (PRL), is organic raw sea salt from prehistoric, unpolluted seabeds. This natural, sun-dried sea salt contains unheated trace minerals in addition to unheated sodium chloride. These minerals, undamaged by heat, retain their high energy, are ideal for helping to maintain fluid balance in the body. Its rich trace mineral content gives it a slightly pink color. It is composed of tiny mineral rich crystals formed millions of years before pollution contaminated our present oceans.

"Rock a Bye Baby" - Sleep

ADHD is linked with a variety of sleep problems. For starters, anyone that is taking an amphetamine should know that your body is artificially stimulated with energy, a fake wake. When the body is stimulated during the day, many children have trouble sleeping because they are so revved up from the drug. Some doctors give children sleeping medications. REALLY? Now we have our children on two toxic drugs.

The National Sleep Foundation "found in one recent study that children with ADHD had higher rates of daytime sleepiness than children without ADHD. Another study found that 50% of children with ADHD had signs of sleep-disordered breathing, compared to only 22% of children without ADHD. Research suggests that restless legs syndrome and periodic leg movement syndrome are also common in children with ADHD."

Anyone that has been around children knows that when children become sleepy, they react by speeding up and overcompensating to avoid sleep unlike adults who just fall asleep. When kids are tired, they become moody, angry, explosive, and aggressive. In another study with 2,463 children with sleep problems, aged 6-15, the children were more likely to be inattentive, hyperactive, impulsive, and display oppositional behaviors. Refer to Chapter 21 for an in-depth study of how to help your kids sleep better.

"Let's Go Out to the Ball Game" - Exercise

A recent study confirms what many parents and educators intuitively realize; physical exercise helps ADHD children function better. The study concludes that physical activity improves cognition, overall improvement in attitude, and in academic skills such as reading and mathematics learning, and has a healthy effect on the brain.

ADHD Research Background

The study, completed by Charles H. Hillman et al., was undertaken over a nine-month period and involved 221 children aged 7 to 9 years. The study was used to see changes in physical fitness, electrical activity in the brain and increases in executive control in the brain (to withstand distractions, remember facts, move from one task to another and increase focus).

Two research studies show the positive links between ADHD and exercise:

#1 - 17 children in Grade 3, four symptoms on the Disruptive Behavior Disorders Rating Scale had 30 minutes of physical activity at school every day for 8 weeks. Between 64% and 71% of the kids showed general improvement.

#2 - 7-year-old children with ADHD, one group had 30 minutes of physical activity (PA) each school day for 12 weeks while the other group was given desk activities. Parents with children that exercised reported their kids were less moody and less inattentive at home."

Exercise raises levels of dopamine and norepinephrine in the brain. These are the feel good neurotransmitters in the brain and are essential for your child's wellbeing. It is important that your child try out different exercises so they can pick the one that resonates with them, not fulfilling a childhood dream of yours or assuming your role. There is nothing worse than trying to live up to your expectations of a sport you were good at. Your child needs to become their own entity, so they can feel good about their achievements. Let them experiment with several sports to find out which one they like the best.

Ideas to help make that perfect match

It is also imperative that you practice with your child to help them feel proud of their achievements. If they do not feel good about the current sport, guide them to find another sport that they may be better at.

> Swimming - Offers: structure and guidance
> Improves: personal development with limited comparison to others: Note: There are many germs/**bacteria in many public pools today**. Chlorine is also a chemical that can seep into our bodies through our skin. Best option is a pool treated with salt!

Martial Arts - Offers: self-control, discipline, and respect. Improves: focus and confidence with step by step instruction.

Tennis - Offers: release of anger or frustration without heavy concentration. Improves: relaxation and release of stress.

Gymnastics - Offers: sense of balance, muscle awareness, core strength. Improves: focus, building muscles, improve sensory processing.

Wrestling - Offers: help for misguided aggression and too much energy. Improves: helps release stress and build positive emotions.

Soccer - Offers: building social skills, friendships. Improves: confidence, constant action to help with short attention spans.

Horseback Riding - Offers: builds relationship and love for animals and to react with calmness instead of harshness, which they learn from the horse. Improves: behavior modification in general.

Track and Cross-Country - Offers: discipline and pacing, team building, limited competition. Improves: self- esteem, social development.

Most exercise will involve a coach that your children will hopefully look up to. However, it is a good idea to see how the coach reacts at games before letting your child sign up for that team. My son was on a team where the coach yelled at many of the team members. What I noticed is that the team reacted in a negative way to the yelling. They seemed to do worse. I approached the coach and suggested taking a different approach to see if the team moral could be improved by complimenting the team and becoming more positive. The conclusion is yes, the team improved with positive results. It is a good idea to let the coach know that your child has ADHD as well as educate and share with them that punishment will not be effective and will only be humiliating and lower your child's self-esteem even more.

"Sugar and Spice and Nothing Nice" - Sugar, Gluten & Soy

Sugar - Although dyes can cause more problems than sugar, kids still have reactions to white sugars, flours, and especially wheat and soy products. There is an easy way to test your child for a sugar reaction. It may be harder than you think because you will need to find a sugar product that has no food dyes. You can make something homemade or give your child a teaspoon or two of sugar and see if their hyperactivity increases. You will need to journal the reaction for the next 2 hours to identify if there are any notable reactions to the sugar. If so, you will know to avoid sugar.

Gluten - It is estimated that one out of every 133 people has Celiac disease or is gluten intolerant. Many people that are gluten intolerant have a much higher risk of having ADHD/ADD. The good news is that once you start your child on a gluten-free diet, you will see significant improvements in your child's hyperactivity, functioning and/or behavior.

Soy - Soy can be another issue since it is hidden in so many products including infant formula, bread and many processed foods. Soy is one of the most heavily pesticide foods because it is a GMO, meaning it requires more pesticides to kill the weeds.

"Bright Colors to Die for" - Dyes, MSG, Artificial Sugars

Another possible alternative is that a child may have an allergy to food dyes or food additives. Americans are now eating 5 times more food dye than in 1955. This reaction can be severe in children who already have other allergies, ear infections, asthma, eczema, sleep disturbances, are unhappy, and have bizarre swings in their mood for no apparent reason. Almost all processed foods contain food coloring and have many unhealthy additives.

"Over the Rainbow" Hidden dangers of food color dyes

Blue #1 Brilliant Blue

Known Dangers: Causes kidney tumors in mice; may induce an allergic reaction in individuals with pre-existing asthma

Commonly found in: baked goods, beverages, candies, cereal

Blue #2 Indigo Carmine

Known Dangers: Causes significant occurrence of tumors, particularly brain gliomas in male rats

Commonly found in: beverages, candies, dog food

Citrus Red #2

Known Dangers: Toxic to rats and mice at modest levels; bladder and other tumors found in mice; labeled "possibly carcinogenic to humans" by the IARC (International Agency for Research on Cancer)

Commonly found in: skin of Florida oranges

Green #3 Fast Green

Known Dangers: As a food dye, it is prohibited in countries that are part of The European Union and some other countries; caused significant increases in bladder tumors in male rats

Commonly found in: beverages, candies, ice cream, cosmetics

Red #40 Allura Red

Known Dangers: Accelerates the appearance of immune system tumors in mice; suspected trigger of hyperactivity in children; causes allergy-like reactions in some people

Commonly found in: beverages, candies, cereal, cosmetics

Red #3 Erythrosine

Known Dangers: Suspected trigger of hyperactivity in children; thyroid carcinogen in animals; partially banned by the FDA in 1990

Commonly found in: baked goods, candies, sausage, maraschino cherries

Yellow #5 Tartrazine

Known Dangers: Can cause allergy-like reactions; may cause mild to severe hypersensitivity reactions; can cause sleep disturbances

Commonly found in: baked goods, candies, cereal, beverages

Yellow #6 Sunset Yellow

Known Dangers: May cause hyperactivity in some children; causes adrenal tumors in animals

Commonly found in: baked goods, sausage, cereal, cosmetics

Many people notice that as soon as they remove dyes from their children's diet their children's symptoms seem to melt away including anger, hyperactivity and an increased comprehension in school with reading, writing and math skills.

There are some great healthy alternatives to artificial dyes including sweet potatoes, beets, pumpkin, carrots, spinach, red cabbage, berries, turmeric and saffron powder. Make sure to purchase Organic products that do not use any artificial dyes; confirm this by thoroughly checking labels.

MSG

MSG (monosodium glutamate) is an excitotoxin. It is a type of neurotoxin that excites your brain cells to death. It can affect a child's mood and behavior, with or without ADHD/ADD. "According to neurosurgeon Russell Blaylock, author of *Excitotoxins: The Taste That Kills*, MSG crosses the blood/brain barrier and can cause the developing nerve fibers to be miswired."

MSG is found in many fast foods (especially Chinese food) and processed foods such as meats, frozen meals, soup mixes, salad dressings, and many others. Be careful when reading labels and looking for MSG under the names of sodium caseinate, autolyzed yeast, and hydrolyzed protein.

If you inject blue dye into the bloodstream, everything turns blue except your brain and spinal cord, protecting your brain. The blood brain barrier

(BBB) only allows some material to cross and shuts the doors to others therefore protecting the brain from foreign substances. The door may be opened by some medications, neurotoxins such as MSG, microwaves, radiation, infections (Lyme), trauma, inflammation and injury to the brain.

Artificial sugar chemicals are not sugars; they are chlorinated sweeteners and very toxic chemicals. The following artificial sweeteners approved by the FDA include acesulfame, aspartame, saccharin, sucralose, and neotame. They are found in diet soda, sugar free candies and cookies. Eliminate all artificial sweeteners.

"I Go Bananas Over Nuts - Eat Sulfur Based Foods"

Sulfur is a mineral that is vital to your health and is found in all body tissues. It plays a crucial role in your health because it helps resist bacteria and protects against toxic substances. Eating a diet high in sulfur has been known to help children with ADHD and ADD. Sulfur foods also help keep our skin, hair and nails looking healthy. Cysteine and methionine are two major sources of sulfur that contain amino acids that serve as enzymes to bring about chemical reactions. Try this wonderful selection of sulfur foods to help reduce ADHD/ADD symptoms.

A gluten and dairy free diet is suggested with those that are ADHD/ADD and to be perfectly honest a good diet for all people. Gluten has been shown to inflame the brain and kill brain cells. Gluten, a protein found in wheat and other grains, is particularly bad if you have ADHD. Research shows that a gluten-free and casein-free diet can significantly decrease ADHD symptoms. Casein is a protein in dairy and removing it from the diet has been shown to improve psychiatric disorders and ADHD symptoms.

"Come Hungry, Leave Happy" Sulfur Based Foods

- Garlic, onions, and all of the allium family
- Grains – gluten free
- Cysteine and methionine are in: sunflower seeds, oats, dark chocolate (very low sugar, not candy), cashews, walnuts, almonds, sesame seeds (in that order). Also, fish and poultry
- Legumes, including carob and jicama
- Eggs
    - of chicken
    - of duck
- Fish and poultry
- Nuts & seeds
- Broccoli, cauliflower and all cruciferous vegetables. This includes cabbages, bok choy, mustard, kale, turnips and watercress.
- Asparagus
- Coconut
- Avocado (high in glutathione, which breaks down during digestion, yielding cysteine)
- Watermelon (also high in glutathione)
- Swiss Chard
- Parsley
- Sweet potatoes and "yams"
- Bananas
- Tomatoes-MSM (Methylsulfonylmethane)
- Tea - (MSM)
- Whey proteins (high in cysteine & methionine)
- Amino acids: cysteine, methionine, thiamin / thiamine / vitamin B1 / aneurine, biotin, vitamin B7 or vitamin H

"Here Comes the Sun" – Get Dirty and Play Outside

The sun is responsible for all life on earth. Plants grow outside in the sun all day and if there are not enough nutrients in the soil and water, the plants will die. The same is true for us. We need the sun and proper nutrients to survive and thrive. We need internal protections instead of toxic sunscreens. Many of us are inside all day. Having the right nutrition is key; so if you are looking to get healthier, take your nutrients and vitamins and get your natural vitamin D outside. Sunlight has been known to help lower blood sugar. Sunlight helps to store the sugar as glycogen in the liver, muscles and cells for later use. Being in the sun also helps stimulate the capillaries, bring blood to the surface, strengthen digestion and improve the eyesight. The sun has also been given credit for helping with hormone balance and we all know it helps with depression and well-being.

Researchers and doctors have blamed the sun for causing cancer. They have gone as far as having our children avoid the sun at all costs. If the sun causes cancer, then why didn't the farmers of thirty years ago get cancer? They were out in the sun all day.

It is my opinion that the sun does not cause cancer; a depressed immune system caused by the intake of toxic chemicals does. I have a lifetime relationship with the sun and worshiped it most of my life. I am now almost 60 and I have no skin cancer. However, I have a superior immune system, have had no colds in 8 years and have healed from 18 different diseases.

I am not telling people to go sit endless hours in the sun. Most people do not have the immune system that can handle it. However, I am not a fan of sunscreen since most of them contain very toxic ingredients. Please see Chapter 20 to learn more about sunscreens. If you work in the sun all day, it is recommended to wear a long sleeve shirt and hat to protect yourself. Allow your skin to absorb ten minutes of sun a day for some natural vitamin D.

Our kids need to play out in the sun and get dirty. I can remember playing kick ball, capture the flag, riding my bike and making mud pies. It is important to take some time each day and let your kids enjoy a little sun when they are over the age of two. Please use common sense and limit your toddler's exposure to the sun by keeping them covered and applying sunscreen without toxic chemicals.

"It Takes Two Hands to Get Rid of this Whopper" - Trans fats

The Top 10 "Trans Fat" Foods to Remove from your Diet

1. Spreads Margarine is a twisted sister -- it is loaded with trans fats and saturated fats, both of which can lead to heart disease. Other non-butter spreads and shortening also contain large amounts of trans fat and saturated fat:
   - Stick margarine has 2.8 grams of trans fat per tablespoon, and 2.1 grams of saturated fat.
   - Tub margarine has 0.6 grams of trans fat per tablespoon, and 1.2 grams of saturated fat.
   - Shortening has 4.2 grams of trans fat per tablespoon, and 3.4 grams of saturated fat.
   - Butter has 0.3 grams of trans fat per tablespoon, and 7.2 grams of saturated fat.

   Best: Pour olive oil in a BPA free plastic container. Add a little pink salt, garlic powder, basil. Put in the freezer. In the morning, transfer to the refrigerator. After using, return to the refrigerator before it turns back to oil.

   Vegan Spreads: Ingredients in these spreads contain **palm and canola oil**. Sorry, I am not a fan. Do not forget when you buy spreads, most are packaged in containers with BPA.
2. Packaged foods Cake mixes, Bisquick, and other mixes all have several grams of trans fat per serving.

   Tip: Add flour and baking powder and make it homemade.
3. Soups Ramen noodles and soup cups contain very high levels of trans fat.

   Tip: Make homemade soups.
4. Fast Food Back away from the fries and chicken and other foods that are deep-fried in partially hydrogenated oil. Even if the chains use liquid oil, fries are sometimes partially fried in trans fat before they are

shipped to the restaurant. Pancakes and grilled sandwiches also have some trans fat from margarine slathered on the grill.

Tip: Order your meat broiled or baked with a baked potato.

5. Frozen Food - Almost all prepackaged foods are made with trans fat. Waffles, pizzas, even breaded fish sticks contain trans fat.
6. Baked Goods - More trans fats are used in commercially baked products such as doughnuts, cookies and cakes.

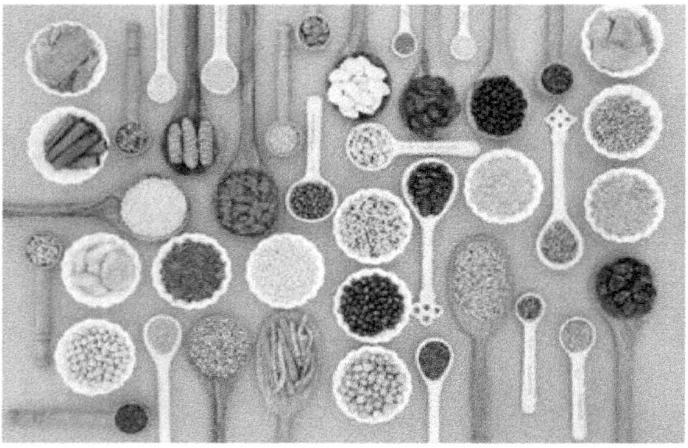

"Just a Spoonful of Supplements Helps Sickness Go Down" – Supplements

Always check with your doctor before starting a supplement program, especially if you are taking medications.

Natural supplements are essential in supporting brain function for kids. A combination of EFA and DHA fatty acids daily with an appropriate balance of omega-3 and omega-6 is key. There are many supplements and combinations to help with ADHD. The following are a list of supplements and amino acids that have shown significant improvement individually in studies to help with the many different issues with ADHD. A comprehensive approach is always necessary. The best way to find the correct supplements for your child is to find a QRA practitioner in your area. This practice is discussed in Chapter 9.

Supplements recommended to help with brain function

1. Ginkgo Biloba - Ginkgo is an ancient plant species and the Ginkgo tree has a long history of medicinal use. Extracts are typically derived from the leaves. It is reported that general memory responses and mental sharpness were improved.
2. Bacopa - monnieri (Brahmi) is an Ayurvedic medicinal herbal preparation that is widely used as a tonic and memory enhancer.
3. Ginseng Korean Red - is a natural stimulant well-regarded for its memory boosting, sleep improving, and brain-saving longevity benefits. It's also known for boosting dopamine and norepinephrine.
4. Siberian ginseng (eleutherococcus senticosus) is a natural brain stimulant that can improve your memory and boost your levels of concentration.
5. Passion Flower- These plant parts contain high amounts of alkaloids, flavonoids and their glycosides. Passion Flower extract was found to provide the same therapeutic benefits for anxiety disorders as oxazepam, a known anxiolytic.
6. Magnesium - Giving them magnesium supplement increased attention span, likely due to this mineral improving brain activity and having a calming effect
7. Zinc - A commonly ignored mineral that can have significant treatment effects on ADHD. Zinc plays an essential role in neurotransmitter function and helps maintain brain health. It is necessary in the metabolism of melatonin, which regulates dopamine.
8. EFA – Omega 3s improve cognitive ability.
9. Iron - 84 percent of children with ADHD had significantly lower levels of iron, compared with 18 percent of kids without ADHD. Too much iron can block the absorption of zinc, copper, and manganese.
10. Valerian - This herbal root may be used to alleviate ADHD symptoms such as anxiety and hyperactivity. Scientists believe that valerian boosts a chemical substance in the brain, which produces a calming effect to treat restlessness, insomnia, and nervousness.

11. Yizhi – A Chinese herbal blend. Yizhi syrup, or wit-increasing syrup, was tested on 66 hyperactive children. Eighty-four percent experienced significant improvement in academic achievement and behavioral ratings, and reduction in other symptoms of ADHD. Urine sample testing showed a significant increase in the neurotransmitters dopamine and norepinephrine.
12. Vitamin D - Vitamin D deficiency has been linked with poor brain health and depression, and because vitamin D interacts with every hormone receptor in the body, it certainly plays a role in attention and hyperactivity. Inadequate vitamin D during pregnancy is linked to fetal brain development problems, autism, and schizophrenia.
13. Greens – super foods, micronutrients, ingredients that come from whole green foods such as kale, spinach, etc. Behavioral disorder, autism and ADHD are greatly affected by nutrition and some children do not get enough vitamins, minerals and enzymes. Powdered greens are a great way to add nutrition into a shake.
14. B Vitamins - B vitamins work together synergistically to support critical functions in the brain. In studies, B-complex has been shown to reduce hyperactivity symptoms and increase serotonin in children with ADHD producing calmer and happier children

Amino Acids to Help With Brain Function

1. Acetyl- L carnitine - Carnitine is necessary for fatty acid metabolism and energy production because it helps remove toxic substances that the body produces. Carnitine is present in all tissues and plays a primary role in brain energy metabolism, influencing neurotransmitter pathways. Carnitine directly enables the brain to process omega-3s.
2. L-Taurine - Taurine works the brain and heart, supports neurological development, and modulates neurotransmitters in the brain. Taurine helps to move minerals such as potassium, sodium, calcium, and magnesium in and out of cells, which generate nerve impulses.

3. Glycine - Glycine is the simplest of the amino acids. It is useful in ADHD therapy for improving memory, attention and mood.
4. L-theanine – This water soluble chemical is in some mushrooms and green tea. It has been shown to enhance your body's antioxidant count, promote mental relaxation, preventing certain forms of cognitive dysfunction and affects the levels of serotonin and dopamine.
5. L-tyrosine- Tyrosine is important in ADHD therapy because it is a precursor of both dopamine and norepinephrine.
6. Methylsulfonylmethane (MSM) - helps to reduce histamine in your body, which is the inflammatory substance responsible for many allergy symptoms

The following is a list of supplements I use and recommend from Premier Research Labs 800-370-3447. I saw a personal transformation in my health, where I had tried many others with no difference; these supplements are very high quality and have helped me to heal. There are other reputable companies, but you must always use the ten requirements for purchasing supplements listed in Chapter 25. If not ordering from Premier Research Labs, I recommend you purchase from a health food store, not from a large discount store. If you do not feel any better with your current supplements, know they most likely do not have a strong enough nutrient value to make a different in your health. If they are cheap or come in a plastic container, do yourself a favor and throw them out.

EPA/DHA

This distinctive oil blend, which includes the use of flaxseed oil, is a premier quality life-essential fatty acid formula for optimal brain and body support, featuring an ideal blend A (gamma linolenic acid) and Omega 3, 6 and 9 essential fatty acids. Premier EFA Oil Blend is comprised of cold-pressed, premier, unrefined oils that are nitrogen-flushed to protect freshness. This blend has a full-bodied gourmet taste that is delicious mixed in food or drinks. This is important for all kids, adults and especially for pregnant women.

DHA

DHA is an essential plant-source that is derived from non-GMO micro-algae instead of fish, making it suitable for everyone including vegetarians and vegans. Feed your brain with plant-source DHA (docosahexaenoic acid), a key Omega-3 fatty acid, important for digestion. This is most important for ADHD/ ADD, Autism, Asthma as well as any other child with health issues.

Max B

Max B is my favorite and I take it every day. Many of my clients feel instant energy from our Max B. The liquid form ensures quick delivery and absorption. Our cells prefer Max B's live source, high energy, end-chain vitamin B forms, over common synthetic (coal tar-derived) sources. This B vitamin-rich formula offers advanced support for the liver, energy, immune system, adrenals and mood balance. Carbohydrates can cause vitamin B deficiencies. Problems associated with B vitamin deficiencies include depression, memory loss, heart disease, insomnia, cataracts, atherosclerosis, fatigue, muscle cramps, allergies and GI symptoms to name just a few. This is great for adults, pregnant women and teens.

AdrenaVen

This product is a must for those with adrenal fatigue. AdrenaVen™ is a premier-quality master formula designed to support healthy adrenal glands, which produce hormones for your organs to function. It features prickly pear, antioxidant qualities and it is also rich in Vitamin C. This is helpful for adults and teens that have low energy. Pregnant women would need to have QRA testing to find out if this would be helpful.

Green Tea ND

Green Tea ND is one of my favorites to help bring energy and healing for those who suffer from a dysfunctional thyroid or just a loss of energy. Green tea leaves are high in polyphenols, which boost the metabolism and help with anti-aging, digestive function, joint flexibility, healthy immune response and rejuvenation support. This is helpful for teens, adults and pregnant women.

Aloe Pro

This organic aloe is not loaded with undesirable preservatives such as sodium benzoate. The pure aloe liquid provides the complete array of aloe's inherent beneficial properties and is unheated. Aloe is high in vitamins, minerals, amino acids and fatty acids. Aloe is a great enhancement for proper digestion for everyone, including kids.

D3

A one-of-a-kind, live-source vitamin D3 delivers cardiovascular and immune system support. Vitamin D3 also aids in calcium absorption for healthy bones and teeth. Recent studies propose ideal vitamin D3 intake should be 2000 IU or more daily (this serum meets the recommendations with just one drop). According to the Office of Dietary Supplements, the recommended dietary allowance, or RDA, for vitamin D in children ages 1 to 19 is 600 IU daily. Premiers D3 is made with extra virgin olive oil; kids, teens and adults all need D3, especially if they are not in the sun.

Pink Sea Salt

Premiers pink sea salt is Unrefined, untreated and unheated. An extract from Mediterranean and Alaea Hawaiian sea and is rich in the trace minerals that children need. A little sea salt each day is a helpful additive for kids, adults, teens and pregnant moms for healthy digestion.

Taurine

Taurine, a sulphur-containing amino acid-like nutrient, is the most abundant free amino acid in the heart and the nervous system. It plays a recognized role in the health of the brain, heart, gallbladder, eyes and the cardiovascular system. Ingredients: Taurine (free form), Lemon Verbena, Aloysia citriodora, Reishi (fruiting body) Ganoderma lucidum, Organic prickly Pear (leaf), Opuntia ficus-ubduca. Individuals should be tested by a QRA Practioner to identify exact dosage but great for adults and teens.

Tyrosine

Tyrosine, a conditionally essential amino acid, is a precursor to the thyroid hormone, thyroxin, and to catecholamine neurotransmitters. Tyrosine also supports your mood during times of occasional stress, when dopamine and norepinephrine levels may need additional support. Ingredients: L-Tyrosine 1,005 mg., Tyro Synergy Support, Rhodiol rosea (root) Extract, Aquamin F Mineralized Red Algae (whole), Turmeric (rhizome) (curcuma longa), Chinese Salvia (root) (Salvia Miltiorrhiza). Great to help with depression, mood and to increase focus. Good for adults, kids and teens. A QRA (Quantitative Risk Assessment) test is recommended. Learn more on QRA testing in Chapter 9.

The following is the Vanderbilt Assessment Scale, which is a test to help parents see if their child is ADHD. MyADHD.com. Vanderbilt Assessment Scale—Parent Informant # 6175.

Name of child:________________Gender:__________Age:__________
Grade:________________________Date: ____________

Completed by: ______________________________
Parent's Phone Number: ______________________

Directions: Each rating should be considered in the context of what is appropriate for the age of your child. When completing this form please think about your child's behavior in the past 6 months.

Is this evaluation based on a time the child __ was on medication __ was not on medication __ not sure?

Never - 0 Occasionally- 1 Often-2 Very Often-3

Symptoms

1. Does not pay close attention to details or makes careless mistakes with, for example, homework

0 1 2 3

2. Has difficulty keeping attention to what needs to be done
0 1 2 3
3. Does not seem to listen when spoken to directly
0 1 2 3
4. Does not follow through on instructions and fails to finish schoolwork, chores, or duties
0 1 2 3
5. Has difficulty organizing tasks and activities 0 1 2 3
6. Avoids, dislikes, or is reluctant to engage in tasks that require sustained mental effort (e.g., schoolwork or homework)
0 1 2 3
7. Loses things necessary for tasks or activities (e.g., toys, school assignments, pencils, books, or tools) 0 1 2 3
8. Is distracted by extraneous stimuli 0 1 2 3
9. Is forgetful in daily activities 0 1 2 3
10. Fidgets with hands or feet or squirms in seat 0 1 2 3
11. Leaves seat in classroom or in other situations in which remaining seated is expected
0 1 2 3
12. Runs about /climbs excessively in situations in which remaining seated is expected
0 1 2 3
13. Has difficulty playing or engaging in leisure activities quietly
0 1 2 3
14. Is "on the go" or often acts as if "driven by a motor"
0 1 2 3
15. Talks excessively 0 1 2 3
16. Blurts out answers before questions have been completed
0 1 2 3
17. Has difficulty waiting in line 0 1 2 3
18. Interrupts or intrudes on others (eg, butts into conversations/games)
0 1 2 3
19. Argues with adults 0 1 2 3

20. Loses temper	0	1	2	3
21. Actively defies or refuses to go along with adult requests or rules	0	1	2	3
22. Deliberately annoys people	0	1	2	3
23. Blames others for his or her mistakes or misbehaviors	0	1	2	3
24. Is touchy or easily annoyed by others	0	1	2	3
25. Is angry or resentful	0	1	2	3
26. Is spiteful and wants to get even	0	1	2	3
27. Bullies, threatens, or intimidates others	0	1	2	3
28. Starts physical fights	0	1	2	3
29. Lies to get out of trouble or to avoid obligations (ie, "cons" others)	0	1	2	3
30. Is truant from school (skips school) without permission	0	1	2	3
31. Is physically cruel to people	0	1	2	3
32. Has stolen things that have value	0	1	2	3
33. Deliberately destroys others' property	0	1	2	3
34. Has used a weapon that can cause serious harm (bat, knife, brick, gun)	0	1	2	3
35. Is physically cruel to animals	0	1	2	3
36. Has deliberately set fires to cause damage	0	1	2	3
37. Has broken into someone else's home, business or car	0	1	2	3
38. Has stayed out at night without permission	0	1	2	3
39. Has run away from home overnight	0	1	2	3
40. Has forced someone into sexual activity	0	1	2	3
41. Is fearful, anxious, or worried	0	1	2	3
42. Is afraid to try new things for fear of making mistakes	0	1	2	3
43. Feels worthless or inferior	0	1	2	3
44. Blames self for problems, feels guilty	0	1	2	3

45. Feels lonely, unwanted, or unloved; complains that "no one loves him or her"	0	1	2	3
46. Is sad, unhappy, or depressed	0	1	2	3
47. Is self-conscious or easily embarrassed	0	1	2	3

<u>Academic Performance</u>

Excellent- 1 Above Average-2 Average-3 Somewhat of a Problem -4 Problematic-5

48. Reading	1	2	3	4	5
49. Mathematics	1	2	3	4	5
50. Written expression	1	2	3	4	5

<u>Classroom Behavioral</u>

Excellent-1 Above Average-2 Average-3 Somewhat a Problem-4 Problematic-5

51. Relationship with peers	1	2	3	4	5
52. Following directions	1	2	3	4	5
53. Disrupting class	1	2	3	4	5
54. Assignment completion	1	2	3	4	5
55. Organizational skills	1	2	3	4	5

Scoring

Total number of items scored 2 or 3 in items 1-9: ______ (ADHD, predominantly inattentive type—6 or more symptoms)

Total number of items scored 2 or 3 in items 10-18:______ (ADHD, predominantly hyperactive-impulsive type—6 or more symptoms)

Total number of items scored 2 or 3 for items 1-18:______ (ADHD, combined type—6 or more symptoms of both types)

Total number of items scored 2 or 3 in items 19-26:______ (oppositional defiant disorder screen—4 or more symptoms)

Total number of items scored 2 or 3 in items 27-40:______ (conduct disorder screen—3 or more symptoms)
Total number of items scored 2 or 3 in items 41-47:______ (anxiety/depression screen—3 or more symptoms)
Scoring Instructions for the Vanderbilt Assessment Scale—Parent Informant

The Vanderbilt Assessment Scale has two components: symptom assessment and impairment of performance.

For the ADHD screen, the symptoms assessment component screens for symptoms that meet the criteria for both inattentive (items 1-9) and hyperactive-impulsive ADHD (items 10-18). To meet DSM-IV criteria for the diagnosis of ADHD, one must have at least 6 responses of "Often" or "Very Often" (scored 2 or 3) to either the 9 inattentive or 9 hyperactive-impulsive items, or both and a score of 4 or 5 on any of the Performance items (48-55). There is a place to record the number of symptoms that meet these criteria in each subgroup.

The Vanderbilt Assessment Scale also contains items that screen for 3 other co-morbidities: oppositional defiant disorder, conduct disorder, and anxiety/depression.

For the oppositional defiant disorder screen there must be a score of 2 or 3 on 4 of the 8 items (19-26) on the subscale and a score of 4 or 5 on any of the Performance items (48-55).

For the conduct disorder screen there must be a score of 2 or 3 on 3 out of the 14 items (27-40) on this subscale and a score of 4 or 5 on any of the Performance items (48-55).

For the anxiety/depression screen there must be a score of 2 or 3 on 3 of the 7 items (41-47) and a score of 4 or 5 on any of the Performance items 48-55).

The Vanderbilt Assessment Scale should NOT be used alone to make a diagnosis. The practitioner must consider information from other sources.

5

"SAVING GOOD HEALTH FROM BAD SCIENCE" - AUTISM

1 out of 68 children and 1 out of 42 Boys

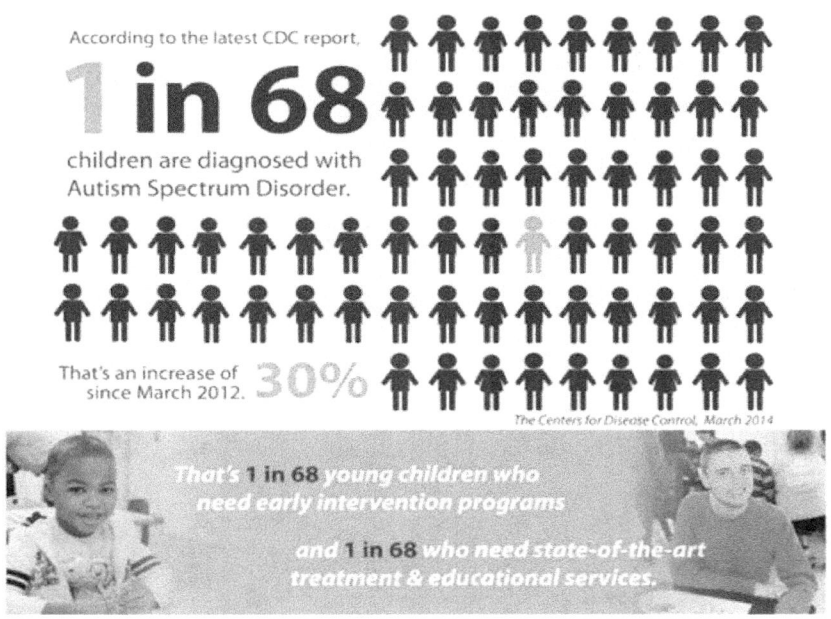

What is Autism?

Autism Spectrum Disorders (ASD) involves five complex, brain-based disorders that affect a person's behavior, social and communication skills. The

Centers for Disease Control describes ASDs as "developmental disabilities that cause substantial impairments in social interaction and communication and the presence of unusual behaviors and interests. Many people with ASDs also have unusual ways of learning, paying attention, and reacting to different sensations. The thinking and learning abilities of people with ASDs can vary—from gifted to severely challenged. An ASD begins before the age of 3 and lasts throughout a person's life." There are four times more boys that have autism than girls.

Autism Spectrum Disorders are characterized by major impairments in social interaction, communication skills, and challenging behaviors. Such behaviors include repetitive motor behaviors (hand flapping, body rocking), resistance to change and, aggression or self-injury. Many individuals with an autism spectrum disorder have above average or average IQ's. 30-50% of people with autism also have seizures.

Five Autism Spectrum Disorders, Pervasive Developmental Disorders (PDD):

- PDD-NOS (Pervasive Developmental Delay – Not Otherwise Specified)
- Autism (sometimes referred to as Classic Autism, Early Infantile Autism, Childhood Autism, or Autistic Disorder)
- Asperger Syndrome
- Rett Syndrome
- Childhood Disintegrative Disorder

Hearing your child has autism is one of the scariest words we could ever hear. It is frightening knowing your life may never be the same for you or your child.

What Causes Autism?

a. **Medical View** - a genetic predisposition, heredity, brain structure
b. **Vaccines View** - studies showing risks for Autism
c. **My hypothesis** - a combination of toxins

1. Already born with toxins that cross the placenta in the womb
2. Chemicals we breathe
3. Foods ingested
4. Vaccines injected
5. Lotions absorbed

Medical Cause of Autism & Treatments

Medical doctors and researchers feel there is no known single cause for autism spectrum disorder. It is theorized that it is caused by abnormalities in brain structure or function, heredity, genetics and medical problems. Brain scans show differences in the shape and structure of the brain in children with autism. Researchers have not found a gene to identify with autism, but they are still searching for irregular segments of genetic code in children that already have Autism. It also appears that some children are born with a susceptibility to autism, but researchers have not yet identified a single "trigger" that causes autism to develop. Researchers are still working on a cluster of unstable genes that may interfere with brain development, viral infections, metabolic imbalances and exposures to chemicals.

Doctors recommend seeking help as soon as you see immature development in your child. They feel that early intervention will help reduce symptoms and speed up your child's development. Doctors have no cure for autism, but offer medications to help with symptoms. Most medications are FDA approved for other conditions such as ADHD, depression, anxiety and sleep disorders. Some people develop tolerance to medications, (when a med stops being effective) or sensitization (when side effects worsen) to medicines.

Medications Used for Autism

a. Selective serotonin re-uptake inhibitors (SSRIs), including fluoxetine is one medication used to help Autism. Even though they are FDA approved for other disorders, they seem to help ease social tension.
b. Naltrexone is FDA-approved for the treatment of alcohol and opioid addictions. It can ease disabling repetitive and self-injurious behaviors in some children with autism.

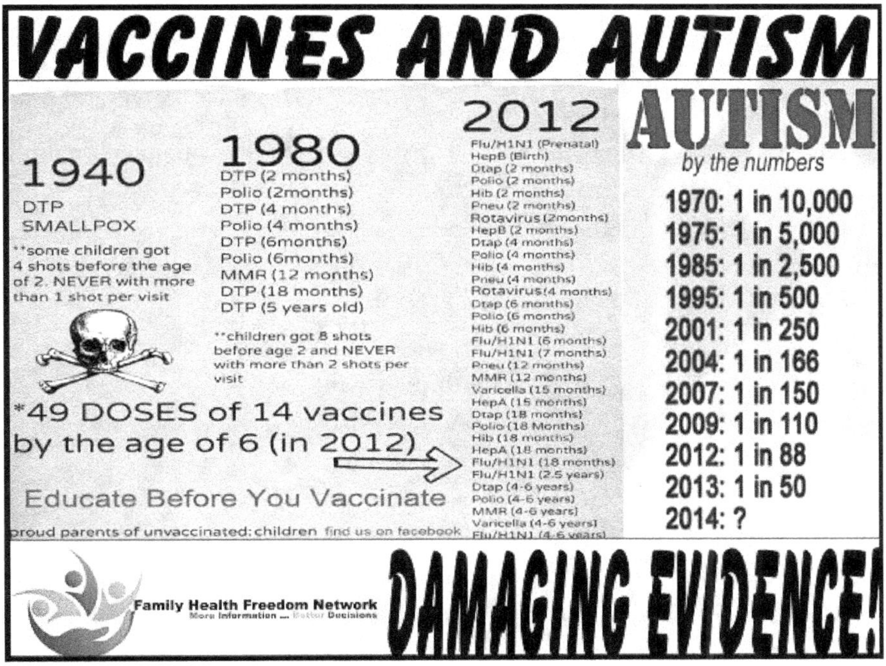
VACCINES AND AUTISM
1940
DTP
SMALLPOX
**some children got 4 shots before the age of 2. NEVER with more than 1 shot per visit
1980
DTP (2 months)
Polio (2months)
DTP (4 months)
Polio (4 months)
DTP (6months)
Polio (6months)
MMR (12 months)
DTP (18 months)
DTP (5 years old)
**children got 8 shots before age 2 and NEVER with more than 2 shots per visit
2012
Flu/H1N1 (Prenatal)
HepB (Birth)
Dtap (2 months)
Polio (2 months)
Hib (2 months)
Pneu (2 months)
Rotavirus (2months)
HepB (2 months)
Dtap (4 months)
Polio (4 months)
Hib (4 months)
Pneu (4 months)
Rotavirus(4 months)
Dtap (6 months)
Polio (6 months)
Hib (6 months)
Flu/H1N1 (6 months)
Flu/H1N1 (7 months)
Pneu (12 months)
MMR (12 months)
Varicella (15 months)
HepA (15 months)
Dtap (18 months)
Polio (18 Months)
Hib (18 months)
HepA (18 months)
Flu/H1N1 (18 months)
Flu/H1N1 (2.5 years)
Dtap (4-6 years)
Polio (4-6 years)
MMR (4-6 years)
Varicella (4-6 years)
Flu/H1N1 (4-6 years)
*49 DOSES of 14 vaccines by the age of 6 (in 2012)
Educate Before You Vaccinate
proud parents of unvaccinated children find us on facebook
AUTISM
by the numbers
1970: 1 in 10,000
1975: 1 in 5,000
1985: 1 in 2,500
1995: 1 in 500
2001: 1 in 250
2004: 1 in 166
2007: 1 in 150
2009: 1 in 110
2012: 1 in 88
2013: 1 in 50
2014: ?
Family Health Freedom Network
DAMAGING EVIDENCE!

Do Vaccines Cause Autism?

You read about it in books and on the internet, watch specials on television and hear about friends of friends that saw a dramatic regressive change in the health of their babies right after they received their vaccines and were shortly diagnosed with autism directly after. The National Vaccine Information Center is a nonprofit educational organization in Vienna, Virginia, run by Barbara Loe Fisher, the parent of an autistic child and co-founder and president. The group was established by the parents of children who were injured or died following vaccination. "They believe that some cases of what Fisher terms the "regressive" form of autism, may be linked to the MMR vaccine. Many organizations around the world have had the same reactions after the vaccines were administered.

Studies Showing Increase Risk of Autism

Universal newborn immunization with hepatitis B vaccine was recommended in 1991. We evaluated the association between hepatitis B vaccination of male neonates and parental report of ASD.

METHODS: This cross-sectional study used U.S. probability samples obtained from National Health Interview Survey 1997-2002 datasets using male boys 3-17 years of age with shot records.

RESULTS: Boys who received the hepatitis B vaccine during the first month of life had **2.94 greater odds for ASD**

CONCLUSION: Findings suggest that U.S. male neonates vaccinated with hepatitis B vaccine had a 3-fold greater risk of ASD; risk was greatest in non-Caucasian boys.

Mercury in the Brain

Environmental Health Perspectives, August 2005 by Thomas Burbacher, PhD [University of Washington]

"This study demonstrates clearly and unequivocally that ethyl mercury, the kind of mercury found in vaccines, not only ends up in the brain, but leaves double the amount of inorganic mercury as methylmercury, the kind of mercury found in fish. This work is groundbreaking because little is known about methylmercury, and many health authorities have asserted that the mercury found in vaccines is the "safe kind. This study also delivers a strong rebuke of the Institute of Medicine's recommendation in 2004 to no longer pursue the mercury-autism connection. This approach is difficult to understand, given our current limited knowledge of the toxic kinetics and developmental neurotoxicity of thimerosal, a compound that has been (and will continue to be) injected in millions of newborns and infants."

See more: http://healthimpactnews.com/2013/30-scientific-studies-showing-the-link-between-vaccines-and-autism/#sthash.D8WOGQdF.dpuf

My Hypothesis – Could Exposure to All Toxins in Combination Cause Autism?

Studies show the following facts

- Today's children are born with cancer causing toxins (287 chemicals were detected in umbilical cord blood from ten babies).
- In 1970, 1 out of every 10,000 children were diagnosed with autism; in 2015, 2015, **1 in 68 children, 1 in 49 boys**.
- Babies are exposed to toxins, (84,000 in existence) in their formula, diapers, cleaning products like bleach, shampoos, lotions, diaper rash ointment, toxic foods: dairy (hormones, antibiotics), fast food, white flour, formaldehyde in tissues, vaccines and napkins.
- Then the "mother lode" is given to our kids in a chemical cocktail of toxins, 49 doses of 14 vaccines by age 6.

Fact: It is now estimated that more than 3.5 million Americans live with autism. The CDC reported in 2014 that about 1 percent of the world population has autism spectrum disorder. (CDC, 2014)

Facts: 287 chemicals were detected in umbilical cord blood from ten babies, 180 cause cancers in humans or animals, 217 are toxic to the brain and nervous system, and 208 cause birth defects or abnormal development in animal tests.

Umbilical Cord Toxic Review

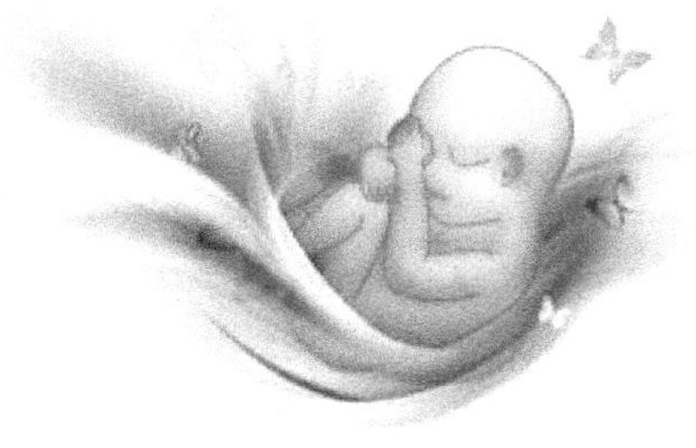

The umbilical cord pulses with at least 300 quarts of blood each day, giving the baby the nutrient and oxygen rich placenta to the rapidly growing child. **"In a study spearheaded by the Environmental Working Group (EWG) in collaboration with Commonweal, researchers at two major laboratories found an average of 200 industrial chemicals and**

pollutants in umbilical cord blood from 10 babies born in August and September of 2004 in U.S. hospitals. Tests revealed 287 chemicals in the group. The umbilical cord blood of these 10 children, collected by Red Cross after the cord was cut, harbored pesticides, consumer product ingredients, and wastes from burning coal, gasoline, and garbage." Environmental Working Group, July 14, 2005

Facts: 1 out of every 3 kids are overweight or obese
1 out of every 10 kids has ADHD
1 out of every 10 has asthma
1 out of every 68 births produce a baby with autism, 1 in 49 boys

Facts: formaldehyde - We eat, breathe and are injected with it from vaccines; formaldehyde is in our napkins, facial tissues, household cleaners, carpet cleaners, disinfectants, medicines, fabric softeners, kid's glues, and antiseptics.

Fact: 49 doses of vaccines injected into children before the age of 6

Facts: Disposable diapers contain some or all of these toxins and they are absorbed through baby's pores. Phythatles, PVC, formaldehyde, alkylphenois, benzend, TEA, MEA, parabens, phosphates, chlorine, chlorinated solvents, ceteareth 20, polyethylene glycol, resorcinol, bronopol, quaternium 15, nanoparticles, triclosan, sulfur oxides, organohides, petrolatum, BPA

Fact: EPA states 84,000 different chemicals are now in use in homes, industry and agriculture

Fact: Chemicals in baby formula copper sulfate and polydextrose

Facts: Researchers view "hygiene hypothesis" as a cause for asthma. (See Chapter 6). Use of sanitizers and a decline in childhood diseases could **depress the immune system** by getting a vaccine instead of the virus.

Coincidence or proof?

Many parents have noticed their children start to have symptoms of autism following vaccination. Evidence shows that there are more toxins in our world; kids are born with toxins, bathed with toxins, fed toxins, breathe toxins and are injected with toxins. It seems relevant to show an astounding increase in cases of Autism

from 1 in 10,000 to 1 in 49, with an increase in the amount of vaccines from 7 in 1970 to 49 in 2016. This compilation of toxins to very young babies from all sources could be the missing link; by depressing their immune systems to the point where a single vaccination combo may cause Autism.

Natural Approach to Autism

The natural approach to Autism is incorporating **everything in this book, especially concentrating on everything in Chapter 4 covering ADHD.** This book is a handbook to incorporate as many healthy choices for the best changes for healing your sick children. The sooner you make them, the better your chances are for improvement to help children heal from diseases. While doctors and researcher believe autism is not something a person simply "grows out of," many natural treatments can help improve symptoms of Autism and now especially, to prevent it. I personally healed from 18 different diseases/disorders naturally, by applying everything in this book. The natural approach involves detoxing the chemicals from the body and putting back in the highest nutrients possible. Autism is a very serious disease; so intense detoxing will be essential. I will recommend finding a QRA practitioner in your area that can help to start with mudpack detoxing for your child's body; this will help pull the toxins out. You can email me personally at heathersholistichealth@yahoo.com for information.

Programs, Assistance & Groups for Autism

ACT Today! SOS is a program dedicated to supporting the immediate and imperative needs of those impacted with autism. ACT Today! Grant Programs established in 2005 do provide access to vital and effective treatments for autism through our quarterly grant cycles. www.act-today.org/SOS

Asperger/Autism Network (AANE) AANE has been given the opportunity, through the generosity of the Doug Flutie Jr. Foundation and private donors, to offer cash grants to those living in New England with Asperger Syndrome. There are two separate programs, one for families of children and one for adults. aane.org

Autism Care and Treatment Today! ACT Today! is a nonprofit 501(c)(3) organization whose mission is to increase access to effective autism treatments. Our goal is to help facilitate treatment by providing the necessary resources including funding, information and referrals to individuals with Autism Spectrum Disorders (ASDs) and their families. www.act-today.org

Autism Consortium: Raising A Child with an ASD All too often, parents of children with ASD incur unexpected and immense out-of-pocket costs for treatments and services. Through the generosity of foundations and, sometimes, public funding, applicable grants might help parents offset these costs. The Autism Consortium has compiled a list of grant opportunities. Be sure to read each option carefully and understand that specific criteria pertain to each. www.autismconsortium.org

Autism Escapes Autism Escapes will serve as an Angel Network for families of children with autism. Its primary purpose is to arrange air travel on private jets for families in need of medical care for their children. www.autismescapes.org

First Hand Foundation is a nonprofit organization that helps children with health-related needs when insurance and other financial resources have been exhausted. Their mission is to directly impact the health status of a young life. applications.cerner.com/firsthand

Friends of Disabled Adults and Children, Too! FODAC is a statewide and national provider of home health care equipment—mobility aids and daily living devices for people with disabilities and the newly injured. www.fodac.org

Fund It Forward is a volunteer run non-profit organization which believes that parents of special needs children are strong, willing and able to endure daily struggles. Their mission is to ease the burdens of families with special needs children by raising money for adaptive equipment not covered by health insurance. www.funditfwd.org

Generation Rescue Family Grant Program This program's grants are designed to provide support to individuals and families affected by Autism Spectrum Disorders. Each grant recipient will receive two doctor visits with a specially trained physician who treats autism; vitamins, minerals and supplements for 90 days; a Generation Rescue mentor; dietary intervention training. generationrescue.org

Helping Hand Program: National Autism Association The Helping Hand Program provides families with financial assistance in getting necessary bio-medical treatments, supplements and therapy services for their autistic child. nationalautismassociation.org

Joey's Fund Family Grant Program accepts grant applications from families in New England (Massachusetts, Connecticut, Rhode Island, Vermont, New Hampshire & Maine) that are in need of financial assistance for their family member(s) with autism. Families can apply for up to $3,000 through the program. You may apply to use the money for anything that directly improves the life of a child with Autism Spectrum Disorder. flutiefoundation.org

Modest Needs is a non-profit organization with a unique, threefold mission: to responsibly provide short-term financial assistance to individuals and families in temporary crisis, to lessen the burden of state and federal agencies charged with the care of the truly indigent by doing everything in their power to stop these at-risk households from slipping into the cycle of poverty, despite the burden posed by an unanticipated, emergency expense; and to promote compassion and generosity on the part of individual persons living in the United States and Canada.www.modestneeds.org

MyGOAL Inc. Enrichment Grant MyGOAL Inc. is proud to offer a grant program that will enable families to take advantage of socialization and educational opportunities designed for individuals with special needs. The purpose of the grants is to enrich the body, mind, and spirit of individual(s) with Autism Spectrum Disorders, resulting in a higher quality of life. mygoalautism.org

Patient Advocate Foundation Find out what is available in your community. Information available on: Children's Health Insurance Programs, Community Referral, Disability Services, Financial Assistance, Food Stamps, Health Care, Insurance, Legal, Medication/Drug Assistance and Special Needs. www.patientadvocate.org

SEAL Naval Special Warfare Family Foundation The NSWKids program supports direct educational diagnostic testing, services and tutoring/mentoring and support to the families of active duty SEALs, SWCC and support personnel who have special needs children. To date, over 100 children and their families have received support. The average cost of care per child is $10,000 depending on the diagnosis and needed services. www.sealnswff.org

Small Steps in Speech assists children with speech and language disorders by funding supplemental therapies and treatments for individuals as well as grants to charitable organizations who serve children with communicative disorders. Their goal is to give children the chance to better express themselves in the world in which we live. www.smallstepsinspeech.org

Talk About Curing Autism: Family Scholarship Program The TACA Family Scholarship Program was developed to help families who are pursuing treatment for their children with autism, but are struggling to find the funding. They understand how difficult it is to stretch the family budget to include things like doctors, independent evaluations or conference registration. It is their desire to provide limited financial assistance to qualified families. tacanow.org

United Healthcare Children's Foundation The United Healthcare Children's Foundation embraces and supports the concept of facilitating access to health-related services that have the potential to significantly enhance either the clinical condition or the quality of life of the child and that are not fully covered by the available commercial health insurance. This support is in the form of a medical grant to be used for medical services not covered or not completely covered by commercial health benefit plans.uhccf.org

Disclaimer - Autism Speaks does not provide medical or legal advice or services. Rather, Autism Speaks provides general information about autism as a service to the community. The information provided on this website is not a recommendation, referral, or endorsement of any resource, therapeutic method, or service provider and does not replace the advice of medical, legal, or educational professionals. Autism Speaks has not validated and is not responsible for any information or services provided by third parties. You are urged to use independent judgment and request references when considering any resource associated with the provision of services related to autism.

Vaxxed - Robert De Niro

Watch these YouTube videos to get current info on vaccines.

https://www.youtube.com/watch?v=EdCU2DfMBpU

https://www.youtube.com/watch?v=FJ7iPn39i08

The following information was taken from the *Vaxxed* site. Robert De Niro did not release the movie because of complications and pressure from groups, producers, etc. Andrew Wakefield, the director, and Del Bigtree, the producer, released a statement, saying, "We were denied due process. We have just witnessed yet another example of the power of corporate interests censoring free speech, art, and truth. Tribeca's action will not succeed in denying the world access to the truth behind the film *Vaxxed*."

"But, many critics had pressured De Niro and the Tribeca Film Festival to drop the film. They argued that by continuing a conversation, especially one sanctioned by such a huge celebrity as De Niro (think how Jenny McCarthy inspired the anti-*Vaxxed* movement), it is legitimizing the anti-vaxxers point of view."

There's a Hole in the Bucket - Leaking a cover up?

"Synopsis – In 2013, biologist Dr. Brian Hooker received a call from a Senior Scientist at the U.S. Centers for Disease Control and Prevention (CDC) who led the agency's 2004 study on the Measles-Mumps-Rubella (MMR) vaccine and its link to autism.

The scientist, Dr. William Thompson, confessed that the CDC had omitted crucial data in their final report that revealed a causal relationship between the MMR vaccine and autism. Over several months, Dr. Hooker records the phone calls made to him by Dr. Thompson who provides the confidential data destroyed by his colleagues at the CDC.

Dr. Hooker enlists the help of Dr. Andrew Wakefield, the British gastroenterologist, falsely accused of starting the anti-vax movement when he first reported in 1998 that the MMR vaccine may cause autism. In his ongoing effort to advocate for children's health, "Wakefield directs this documentary examining the evidence behind an appalling cover-up committed by the government agency charged with protecting the health of American citizens. Interviews with pharmaceutical insiders, doctors, politicians, and parents of vaccine-injured children reveal an alarming deception that has contributed to the sky-rocketing increase of autism and potentially the most catastrophic epidemic of our lifetime."

Tips for Parents

The following are skills, support and suggestions for the right type of treatment plan if your child has autism to help them function in society and at home.

1. Educate yourself on the pros and cons so you can make an informed decision as to how to proceed with treatment.
2. Find what triggers your child and explore with professionals (counselors, teachers, and resource books) what and how to handle them.
3. Review Chapter 11 on relaxation techniques and explore to see which are suitable and will work for your child. Many children with autism are hypersensitive or under-sensitive to light, sound, touch, taste, and smell. Figure out what sensations trigger your child's "bad" or disruptive behaviors and what elicits a positive response.
4. Express your love to your child. This is critical and one of the most helpful expressions for autistic child. Accept them for who they are.
5. Take time outs for yourself. Having an Autistic child can be one of the most stressful conditions; you may often feel overwhelmed, stressed, or discouraged. Make sure to find sitters so you can go out and relax by a quiet dinner, a massage, etc.
6. Safety is top priority. You will need to explore options to keep them safe at all times. Join groups or talk with others that have autistic kids and find out what works best for you.
7. Be patient and consistent. Children need routines to feel safe and comfortable. What is done at school should be also done at home staying with the same structured schedule for learning, meals, bedtime, etc.
8. Use a reward system with praise for good behavior. Try not to make rewards with unhealthy food as autistic children react negatively to

sugary treats. Good healthy food is your best friend when treating autism.

9. Create a private space in your home where they can relax and feel safe. Labeling an area with colored tape or blocks as an area to stay in can be fun for them and be their "go to" safe haven.
10. Find your way to communicate with them through talking, body language or sign language. Find the best way, even if your child is unable to talk; learn their silent language through gestures, sounds, facial expressions, etc.
11. Plan fun activities with your child. Outdoor playtime will help them to burn off some extra energy, providing them with some relaxation and fun.

A Good Autism Treatment Plan

Build on your child's interests, needs and strengths. Know their weaknesses to help identify things that will not work as well. Keep it simple with easy steps and a reward system. Incorporate time for relaxing or having fun with another activity.

Provide regular reinforcement of behavior and focus on reducing problematic behaviors. Build on communication, social skills, sensory problems, motor skills, and emotional issues.

Treatments include - behavior therapy, speech-language therapy, play-based therapy, physical therapy, occupational therapy, and nutritional therapy. Joining a support group is a great way to meet others facing the same challenges. It can also be a great way to set up play time with other kids and to get the emotional support you need.

Counseling for you, your child, and the entire family can be very helpful.

Government Grants and Assistance

Under the U.S. federal law, known as the Individuals with Disabilities Education Act (IDEA), children with disabilities—including those with Autism Spectrum Disorders—are eligible for a range of free or low-cost services. Under this provision, children in need and their families may receive medical evaluations, psychological services, speech therapy, physical therapy, parent counseling and training, assistive technology devices, and other specialized services.

Children under the age of 10 do not need an autism diagnosis to receive free services under IDEA. If they are experiencing a developmental delay (including delays in communication or social development), they are automatically eligible for early intervention and special education services.

Infants and toddlers through the age of two receive assistance through the Early Intervention program. In order to qualify, your child must first undergo a free evaluation. If the assessment reveals a developmental problem, you will work with early intervention treatment providers to develop an Individualized Family Service Plan (IFSP). An IFSP describes your child's needs and the specific services he or she will receive.

For autism, an IFSP would include a variety of behavior, physical, speech, and play therapies. It would focus on preparing autistic kids for the eventual transition to school. Early intervention services are typically conducted in the home or at a child care center.

Ask your pediatrician for a referral.

Autism Special Education Services

Children over the age of three receive assistance through school-based programs. As with early intervention, special education services are tailored to your child's individual needs. Children with Autism Spectrum Disorders are often placed with other developmentally delayed kids in small groups where they can receive more individual attention and specialized instruction. However, depending on their abilities, they may also spend at least part of the school day in a regular classroom. The goal is to place kids in the least restrictive environment possible where they are still able to learn.

If you would like to pursue special education services, your local school system will first need to evaluate your child. Based on this assessment, an Individualized Education Plan (IEP) will be created. An IEP outlines the educational goals for your child for the school year. Additionally, it describes the special services or aids the school will provide your child in order to meet those goals.

6

"I CAN'T HUFF OR PUFF OR BLOW YOUR HOUSE DOWN" ASTHMA

Asthma Attacks Among Persons with Current Asthma — United States, 2001-2010 from the CDC

- Number of children, under 18, who currently have asthma: 6.3 million. 8.6% more boys have asthma than girls
- Number of adults currently with asthma: 17.7 million. 7.4% more women have asthma than men.
- Number of visits to physician offices with asthma as primary diagnosis: 10.5 million
- Number of visits to emergency departments with asthma as primary diagnosis: 1.8 million
- Hospital inpatient care Number of discharges with asthma as first-listed diagnosis: 439,000. Average length of stay: 3.6 days
- Mortality Number of deaths: 3,630

The Medical View of Asthma

An article from the National Institute of Health (NIH)

- How can asthma be prevented? "You can't prevent asthma"
- What is the exact cause of asthma? The exact cause of asthma is unknown

"Researchers think some genetic and environmental factors interact to cause asthma, most often early in life." These factors include:

a. An inherited tendency to develop allergies, called atopy (AT-o-pe)
b. Parents who have asthma
c. Certain respiratory infections during childhood and eczema (an allergic skin condition)
d. Contact with some airborne allergens or exposure to some viral infections in infancy or in early childhood when the immune system is developing
e. "Hygiene Hypothesis"
    a. "Indoor fungus or a large amount cockroaches predispose asthma." **Also exposure to someone that is smoking in the same area as small kids.**
    b. One theory researchers have for what causes asthma is the "hygiene hypothesis." "They believe that our Western lifestyle—with its emphasis on hygiene and sanitation—has resulted in changes in our living conditions and an overall decline in infections in early childhood." **This makes sense because children used to play outside getting exposure to the elements: sun, dirt and fresh air, even drinking out of the hose. Today's kids play indoor games, use sanitizers, and just don't get dirty.**
    c. "Many young children no longer have the same types of environmental exposures and infections as children did in the past. This affects the way that young children's immune systems develop during very early childhood, and it may increase their risk for atopy and asthma." **Kids that grew up in the 50's and 60's would catch the actual infecious diseases such as chicken pox, mumps and measles; these may have strengthened the immune system and they received less vaccines.**
    d. Occupational asthma. - Some people develop asthma because of contact with certain chemical irritants or industrial dusts in the workplace. **This may be due to the existence of 86,000**

toxins in the United States. Today, babies are exposed to toxins through diapers, formula, vaccines, tissues, cleaning products, creams, medications, and more; all at a very early age.

Common signs and symptoms of asthma include:

1. Coughing is worse at night or early in the morning
2. Wheezing, a whistling that occurs when you breathe
3. Chest tightness feels like something is sitting on your chest
4. Shortness of breath, can't catch their breath or out of breath
5. A runny nose
6. Swollen nasal passage
7. Allergic skin conditions (such as eczema)
8. Some kids will have asthma with none of these symptoms
9. Sinus problems
10. Small airways that become even narrower during colds or respiratory infections

What Triggers Asthma Symptoms To Occur?

1. Allergens from animal fur, cockroaches, dust, mold, and pollens from trees, grasses, and flowers
2. Irritants such as cigarette smoke, air pollution, chemicals or dust in the workplace, compounds in home décor products, and sprays (such as hairspray)
3. Medicines such as aspirin or other nonsteroidal anti-inflammatory drugs and nonselective beta-blockers
4. Sulfites in foods and drinks
5. Viral upper respiratory infections, such as colds
6. Physical activity - exercise can be a trigger but talk with your doctor to see if you can still enjoy an active life, which can boost your immune system and keep you healthy.

Physical Exam

Your doctor will listen to your breathing and look for signs of asthma or allergies. They will look at your medical history along with a physical exam and some of or all of the tests listed below. Your doctor will also determine the severity of your asthma: intermittent, mild, moderate, or severe. The level of severity will define what treatment will be recommended. Severe symptoms can be fatal. It's important to treat symptoms when you first notice them. Asthma is different for every child but with proper treatment, most will have few symptoms at night and during the day. Most children who have asthma develop their first symptoms before the age of 5, but it is also hard to diagnose asthma in kids 0 to 5 years of age.

Diagnostic Tests

Lung Function Test

Your doctor will use a test called spirometry (spi-ROM-eh-tre) which checks how your lungs are working and measures how much air you can breathe in and out and how fast you can blow air out.

Allergy testing

A test to measure how sensitive your airways are. This is called a bronchoprovocation (brong-KO-prav-eh-KA-shun) test. Using spirometry, this test repeatedly measures your lung function during physical activity or after you receive increasing doses of cold air or a special chemical to breathe in.

Addiontional Tests

Your doctor may order tests for reflux disease, vocal cord dysfunction, or sleep apnea; all of which have some of the same symptoms as asthma.

An EKG

Eelectrocardiogram or chest X-ray to check for a foreign object or other diseases.

How Is Asthma Treated and Controlled?

Asthma is a long-term disease that doctors and researchers feel has no cure. Their goal of asthma treatment is to control the disease with medication.

- Asthma is treated with two types of medicines: long-term control and quick-relief medicines. Long-term control medicines help reduce airway inflammation and prevent asthma symptoms. Quick-relief, or "rescue," medicines relieve asthma symptoms that may flare up quickly.
- Your level of asthma may worsen if exposed to environmental toxins in your home, school or work.
- You may need more than one kind of medicine or higher doses of medicine to control your asthma.
- Asthma medications can be taken in pill form, but most are taken using a device called an inhaler. An inhaler allows the medicine to go directly to your lungs.

Long-Term Control Medicines

Inhaled corticosteroids are the preferred treatment for young children. Montelukast and cromolyn are other options. Treatment might be given for a trial period of 1 month to 6 weeks. It helps reduce inflammation and swelling that makes your airways sensitive to certain inhaled substances.

Doctors and researcher have an opinion that "Inhaled corticosteroids generally are safe when taken as prescribed. These medicines are different from the illegal anabolic steroids taken by some athletes. Inhaled corticosteroids are not habit-forming, even if you take them every day for many years." Others feel any medication, especially any type of corticosteroids, can form a dependency and are very dangerous if coming off of this medication. Always seek doctor's advise, and never discontinue a medication unless following doctors orders.

If you have severe asthma, you may have to take corticosteroid pills or liquid for short periods to get your asthma under control.

<u>Cromolyn</u>

This medicine is taken using a device called a nebulizer. As you breathe in, the nebulizer sends a fine mist of medicine to your lungs. Cromolyn helps prevent airway inflammation.

<u>Omalizumab</u> (anti-IgE)

This medicine is given as a shot (injection) one or two times a month. It helps prevent your body from reacting to asthma triggers, such as pollen and dust mites. Anti-IgE might be used if other asthma medicines have not worked well.

A rare, but possibly life-threatening allergic reaction called anaphylaxis might occur when the Omalizumab injection is given.

Inhaled long-acting beta2-agonists

These medicines open the airways. They might be added to inhaled corticosteroids to improve asthma control. Inhaled long-acting beta2-agonists should never be used on their own for long-term asthma control. They must be used with inhaled corticosteroids.

Leukotriene modifiers

These medicines are taken by mouth. They help block the chain reaction that increases inflammation in your airways.

Theophylline

This medicine is taken by mouth. Theophylline helps open the airways. With some medicines, like theophylline, your doctor will check the level of medicine in your blood. This helps ensure you are getting enough medicine to relieve your asthma symptoms, but not so much that it causes dangerous side effects.

Quick-Relief Medicines

- Inhaled short-acting beta2-agonists are the first choice for quick relief.
- These medicines act quickly to relax tight muscles around your airways when you're having a flareup. This allows the airways to open up so air can flow through them.
- You should take your quick-relief medicine when you first notice asthma symptoms. If you use this medicine more than 2 days a week, talk with your doctor about your asthma control. You may need to make changes to your asthma action plan.
- Carry your quick-relief inhaler with you at all times in case you need it. If your child has asthma, make sure that anyone caring for him or her has the child's quick-relief medicines, including staff at the child's school. They should understand when and how to use these medicines and when to seek medical care for your child.

- You should not use quick-relief medicines in place of prescribed long-term control medicines. Quick-relief medicines don't reduce inflammation.

Use a Peak Flow Meter

This small, hand-held device shows how well air moves out of your lungs. You blow into the device and it gives you a score, or peak flow number. Your score shows how well your lungs are working at the time of the test. Your peak flow meter can help warn you of an asthma attack, even before you notice symptoms.

Emergency Care – Get to the Hospital If you have Worsening Symptoms

- You have trouble walking and talking because you are out of breath
- You have blue lips or fingernails
- You are having trouble getting air into your lungs

Side Effects

- Inhaled corticosteroids can possibly slow the growth of children of all ages. Slowed growth usually is apparent in the first several months of treatment, is generally small, and doesn't get worse over time.
- Sore mouth, sore throat, or hoarseness
- Cough and spasms of the large airways (bronchi)
- Decreased bone thickness in adults
- Clouding of the lens of the eye (cataract)
- Side effects from inhaled corticosteroids is a mouth infection called thrush. You might be able to use a spacer or holding chamber on your inhaler to avoid thrush and be sure to rinse your mouth out.

Pregnant Women

Pregnant women who have asthma need to control the disease to ensure a good supply of oxygen to their babies. Poor asthma control increases the risk of preeclampsia, a condition in which a pregnant woman develops high blood pressure and protein in the urine. Poor asthma control also increases the risk that a baby will be born early and have a low birth weight.

Studies show that it's safer to take asthma medicines while pregnant than to risk having an asthma attack.

Talk with your doctor if you have asthma and are pregnant or planning a pregnancy. Your level of asthma control may get better or it may get worse while you're pregnant. Your health care team will check your asthma control often and adjust your treatment as needed.

The Holistic Approach to Asthma

As always, the natural or holistic approach to asthma is quite the opposite. As you know, the premise of this book is to heal or reverse disease, which I have successfully healed from 18 different diseases/disorders. In contrast to medical beliefs, I totally believe that asthma and other diseases are not only preventable but curable as well. Our twins both had asthma as children; but today, both have no current symptoms and haven't in 6 or more years.

Please make sure you read Chapter 4 on ADHD in its entirety as it covers a lifestyle to help everyone heal from disease, including asthma. I have worked with many people that have lung diseases/issues from COPD, bronchitis, asthma and upper respiratory issues. I use the mud pack detox system which is very successful. The clay process is discussed in the Chapter 25 on how to detox. This is one of the most powerful ways to detox toxins out of the body, including the lungs. In addition to the mud packing, I also suggest purchasing supplements from Premier Research Labs. This company rates one of my highest scores for quality and effectiveness, scoring a 10 out of 10. Make sure to read Chapter 25 to learn the essential 10 requirements for safe and effective supplement recommendations. These 3 supplements are recommended for a holstic approach to healing/treating asthma:

- Pnemo (improve lung function)
- Aller caps (open up air passages)
- Nucleoimmune (to remove infection)

The first step is removing the toxicity from the lungs (mud pack detox). Then adding the three supplements listed above to kill the infection, make breathing easier and giving essential nurishment to the lungs, helping them to heal. This process has helped to bring back the sense of smell, easier breathing, removal of infection, and helping people with chronic lung issues. Always consult with your doctor while using holistic supplements. Never detox off any medication without a doctors help and/or suggestion.

The following are herbal suggestions/home remedies that may help with asthma

1. Ginger is a well-known natural treatment for various ailments including asthma. Researchers have found that it can help reduce airway inflammation and inhibit airway contraction. Cut one inch of ginger into small pieces and add it to a pot of boiling water. Let it steep for five minutes, allow it to cool down and then drink it. You can also eat raw ginger mixed with salt.
2. Rubbing peppermint essential oils on your temples, under your nose, and chest to help open up the airways. Do this several times a day until the symptoms subside.
3. Figs promote respiratory health, help drain phlegm and alleviate breathing difficulties.
   Wash three dried figs and soak them in a cup of water for several hours. They are very sweet so most kids will love them. Eat the figs and drink the water on an empty stomach.
4. Garlic fights infection and can clear congestion. Boil two or three cloves in one-quarter cup of water. Allow it to cool to room temperature and then drink it. Also eat garlic in foods often.
5. Organic Coffee for adults only - The caffeine in regular coffee can help control asthma attacks because it acts as a bronchodilator. Hot coffee helps relax and clear the airways to help you to breathe easier. The stronger the coffee, the better the result. Not recommended for children. Drink only an 8 oz. cup per day, in the morning hours.

6. Eucalyptus Oil - Pure eucalyptus essential oil acts as a decongestant. Research indicates that it has a chemical called eucalyptol which can help break up mucus. Add a few drops to a cup of hot water and breathe deeply. Buy a vaporizer or one of the new diffusers and add a few drops. Helps to add moisture and scent into the air.

7

"KHEMICAL KIDS" – MEDICATIONS AND VACCINATIONS

First, we need to look at the worldwide statistics, which clearly show that more babies die in the U.S. than any other industrialized country. How can one of the **greatest countries in the world have the worst mortality rates for our babies**?

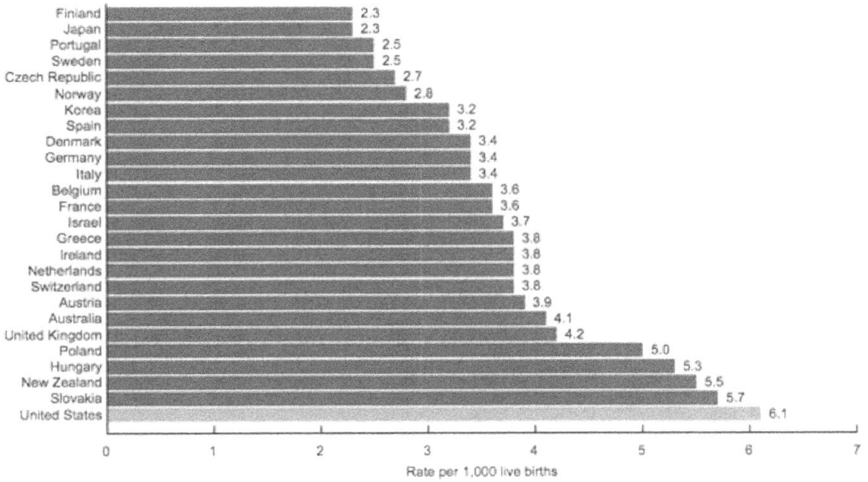

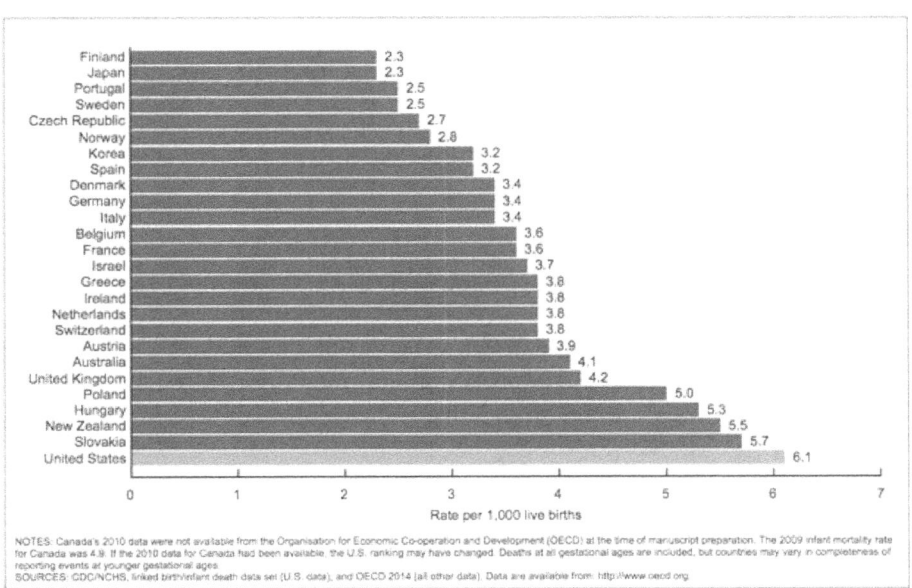

NOTES: Canada's 2010 data were not available from the Organisation for Economic Co-operation and Development (OECD) at the time of manuscript preparation. The 2009 infant mortality rate for Canada was 4.9. If the 2010 data for Canada had been available, the U.S. ranking may have changed. Deaths at all gestational ages are included, but countries may vary in completeness of reporting events at younger gestational ages.
SOURCES: CDC/NCHS, linked birth/infant death data set (U.S. data), and OECD 2014 (all other data). Data are available from: http://www.oecd.org

Medications

Medications came into existence in the United States around 1865. Before that there were healers, aka witches (I resemble that) that used natural/herbal plants to treat people. In the 1930's medications or synthetic drugs replaced the herbal treatments. A synthetic drug is a chemical or biological reaction involving two or more simpler substances in a lab to produce a drug usually not derived from plants. Medications are usually much stronger than herbals treatments and pose more of a danger than that of herbal supplements.

2012 – 2013 leading causes of death:

Heart disease: 611,105
Cancer: 584,881
Chronic lower respiratory diseases: 149,205
Accidents (unintentional injuries): 130,557
Stroke (cerebrovascular diseases): 128,978
Alzheimer's disease: 84,767
Diabetes: 75,578
Influenza and Pneumonia: 56,979
Nephritis, nephrotic syndrome, and nephrosis: 47,112
Intentional self-harm (suicide): 41,149

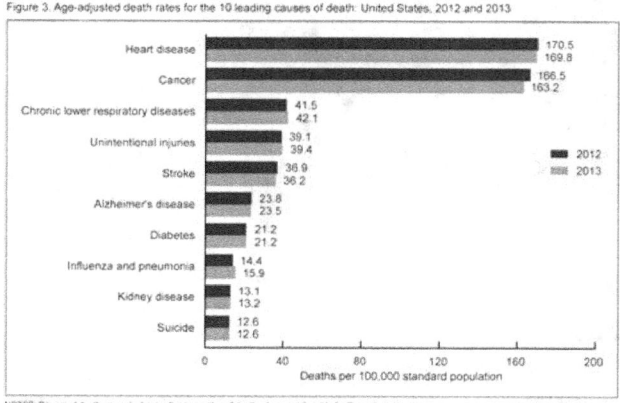

Figure 3. Age-adjusted death rates for the 10 leading causes of death: United States, 2012 and 2013

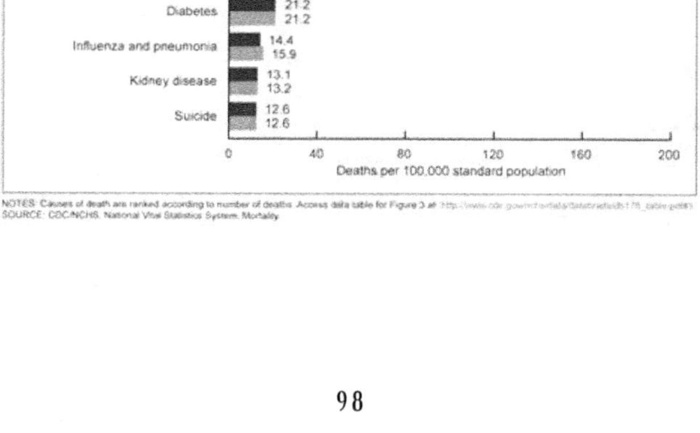

NOTES: Causes of death are ranked according to number of deaths. Access data table for Figure 3 at [illegible]
SOURCE: CDC/NCHS, National Vital Statistics System, Mortality.

How Medical Errors and Prescription Drugs Kill 1 Million People a Year

The International Counsel of Truth in Medicines is a panel of medical doctors, Carolyn Dean MD ND, Martin Feldman MD, Debora Rasio MD, Dorothy Smith PhD, Gary Null PhD. Each have different statistics. They wrote an article called Death by Medicine: How Medical Errors and Prescription Drugs Kill 1 Million People a Year. Below is just a portion of the statistics from their study. Their studies include over 150 references, many from the FDA and CDC.

"A definitive review and close reading of medical peer-review journals, and government health statistics shows that American medicine frequently causes more harm than good. The number of people having in-hospital, adverse drug reactions (ADR) to prescribed medicine is 2.2 million.

- Dr. Richard Besser, of the CDC, in 1995, said the number of unnecessary antibiotics prescribed annually for viral infections was 20 million. Dr. Besser, in 2003, now refers to **tens of millions of unnecessary antibiotics**.
- The number of unnecessary medical and surgical procedures performed annually is 7.5 million.
- The number of people exposed to unnecessary hospitalization annually is 8.9 million.
- The total number of iatrogenic (illness caused by medical examination or treatment) deaths is 783,936.
- In the United States there are greater than four million visits to the emergency departments, to doctors' offices, and to other outpatient settings due to medication-related injury.

Currently, herbs are much less expensive than their human-made counterparts are. The average prescription drug price is about $50 for a month's supply. Herbals cost between $10 and $20 per month per supplement. Total sales of herbs in the U.S. in 2000 were $16 billion compared to $130 billion for outpatient prescription drugs.

"Bet you Can't Eat Just One" Legal Drugs

Did you EVER hear of someone healing from Heart Disease or Diabetes from taking medications? People on medications will take their medications to their grave. Medical doctors learn in medical school how to do surgery, remove organs and to prescribe medications. Medications are only a Band-Aid, a temporary way to treat only symptoms and relieve pain. However, medical doctors are essential for life threatening accidents and all acute situations. The medical doctors treat the symptoms, not cure the problems. If you get an UTI, you take an antibiotic, which will get rid of the infection right? Well, yes, but only temporarily. Most people will get the same infection again. Why? The toxicity will come out in different locations in the body, or different organs, most likely where an organ is more deficient or toxic. Remember the original problem still has not been addressed. People will need to detox their bodies with supplements, improve their diets and detox those organs that are toxic.

Are the medications you are taking making you worse? Did you know that alcohol is a drug? "Say no to drugs," Users are losers," there is no difference between illicit drugs and prescription drugs. Medications make your immune system even more depressed, causing more internal infections, squashing your energy and making your body even weaker. The greatest cause of death, following a successful surgery is secondary infection. With a depressed immune system, secondary infections are deadly. The danger is that almost all medications are used forever/permanently and they are altering and changing your body's natural functions. "Riddle Me This" Has your doctor ever taught you how to live healthy with diet, vitamins, enzymes and minerals?

If you are currently taking any type of medication, never detox yourself. Instead make an appointment with your doctor to follow the proper instructions for your detox. I recommend healing your body first with the life changing therapies in this book before you ever think of getting off of your medications. Most of you will heal and the proof will be the blood test results from your doctor telling you that you no longer need medication. Happy Dance!

"Day off Diet" Results – Food Heals

I currently help with a Facebook page of over 7,000 people, the "Dr. Oz Day off Diet." This is a great detox diet and shows people how to prepare and eat homemade foods, eliminating all the junk in their diets. I did a survey and 20 people reported that they had eliminated one or more prescription drugs from being on the "Day off Diet" in just 4 months.

How did I get sick? "Let me count the ways"

- Smoking
- Medications
- Drugs
- Alcohol
- Stress
- Surgeries
- Bad teeth
- Mercury fillings
- Poor mental health
- Eating meats
- Dairy products
- Pesticides
- Antibiotics
- Junk foods
- Sugar
- Eating out
- Eating fast food
- White flour products
- Caffeine: coffee & sodas

"If you continue to do what you have always done, you will continue to develop what you have created." POOR HEALTH!

Prescription medication is part of daily life for millions of people worldwide. In fact, most people put all of their trust in their medical doctors, to lead them down the path to health. It has been stated that when medications are used in accordance with medical guidelines, they can maintain health and sustain life. This is true, but nothing is stated about healing from these diseases or disorders. It is not just prescription medications that are abused; many illegal drugs such as cocaine, amphetamines, heroin and many legal drugs such as alcohol and nicotine are abused as well.

Over 100,000 people die each year from prescription drug side effects in the U.S. alone. This does NOT include deaths from doctors accidentally prescribing the wrong drugs, pharmacists filling the prescription incorrectly, or from patients overdosing. Researchers have estimated that medications cause 17 million visits to emergency rooms and 8.7 million hospitalizations each year. Medicines are one of the leading causes of death in America, so it becomes imperative for physicians, pharmacists and patients to be aware of those drugs that are most likely to cause problems and in certain circumstances even death.

Drugging America – The Big Bucks

Washington D.C., March 27, 2011 – Pharmaceuticals are a $650 plus billion dollars a year industry. For years, the most profitable business in the U.S. has been the pharmaceutical corporations, which routinely top the annual Fortune 500 list. Doctors prescribe drugs to support an industry, which out-earns the Gross National Product, (GNP) of many nations. America scores highest with people taking over two or more prescriptions a day. Sad statistics.

A new study from York University on January 7, 2008 "estimates the U.S. pharmaceutical industry spends almost twice as much on promotion as it does on research and development, contrary to the industry's claim. The U.S. pharmaceutical **industry spent 24.4% of the sales dollar in 2004 on promotion, versus 13.4% for research and development,** as a percentage of US domestic sales of US $235.4 billion."

Why are they advertising Drugs on Television?

Why are they? Did you know that drug companies spend over 5 billion dollars in drug advertising a year? When advertising a product, the ultimate purpose is for that item to make money. The pharmaceutical companies are so "in our faces," and their drug sales and profits are up. The drugs may be legal, but the drugs do the same thing to your body that the illegal drugs do, they lower your immune system. Sure people are living longer, but with what quality of life?

It is no surprise that the US scores the highest in the world, showing that Americans take on average, 2.2 prescriptions per person.

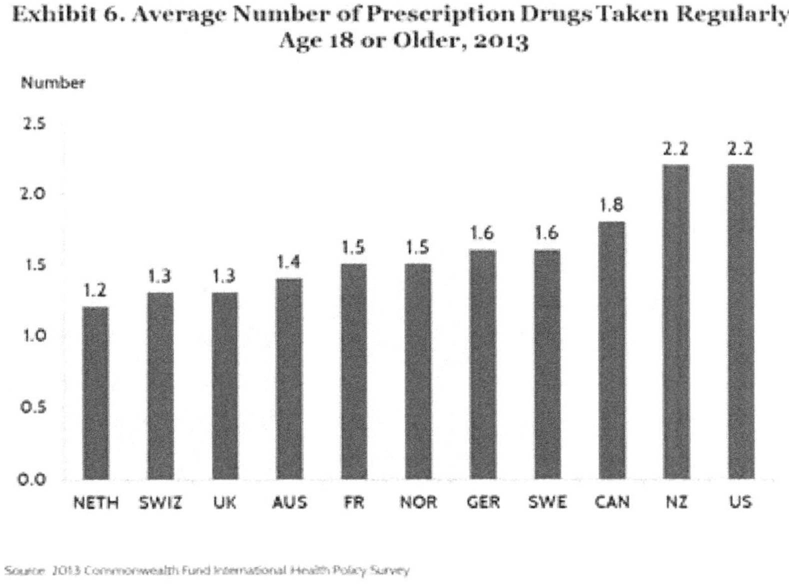

Vaccinations

What are vaccines?

Here is a definition of vaccines from a federal government website managed by the U.S. Department of Health and Human Services named vaccines.gov

- "A vaccine is a product that produces immunity from a disease and can be administered through needle injections, by mouth, or by aerosol.
- A vaccination is the injection of a killed or weakened organism that produces immunity in the body against that organism.
- An immunization is the process by which a person or animal becomes protected from a disease. Vaccines cause immunization, and there are also some diseases that cause immunization after an individual has recovered from the disease."

Why the Government Wants Kids Vaccinated

More than ten million vaccines are administered to children under one-year-old and usually between 2 and 6 months. The FDA states that this is the time where infants are at risk for medical illnesses and serious infant diseases such as: sudden infant death syndrome (SIDS), cancers, heart disease, asthma, seizures, fevers, and more. Although some infants coincidentally have an adverse reaction shortly after a vaccine, the FDA states it does not conclude that the vaccines caused the event. They instead report, this event should be studied further in a "controlled fashion."

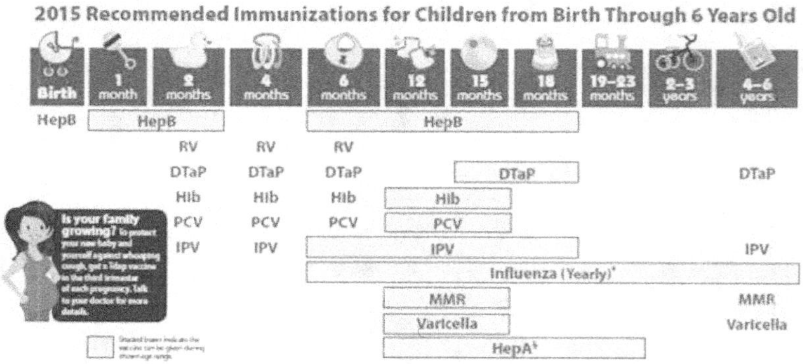

Explore this site from the CDC to look at ALL the Ingredients for Vaccines

http://www.cdc.gov/vaccines/pubs/pinkbook/downloads/appendices/B/excipient-table-2.pdf

Additives used in the production of vaccines may include

1. Suspending fluid (e.g. sterile water, saline, or fluids containing protein)
2. Preservatives and stabilizers to help the vaccine remain unchanged (Albumin, phenols, and glycine)
3. Adjuvants or enhancers to help the vaccine to be more effective

Common substances found in vaccines include:

1. Aluminum gels or salts of aluminum are added to help the vaccine stimulate a more potent, earlier, and more persistent immune response.
2. Antibiotics are added to some vaccines to prevent the growth of germs (bacteria) during production and storage of the vaccine. No vaccine produced in the United States contains penicillin (always check with your doctor or pharmacist to be sure).
3. Egg protein is found in both influenza and yellow fever vaccines, which are prepared using chicken eggs (always check with your doctor or pharmacist to be sure).
4. Formaldehyde is used to inactivate bacterial products for toxoid vaccines and to kill unwanted viruses and bacteria that might contaminate the vaccine during production. Most formaldehyde is removed from the vaccine before it is packaged.
5. Monosodium glutamate (MSG) and 2-phenoxy-ethanol which are used as stabilizers in a few vaccines to help the vaccine remain unchanged when the vaccine is exposed to heat, light, acidity, or humidity.
6. Thimerosal is a mercury-containing preservative that is added to vials of vaccine that contain more than one dose to prevent contamination and growth of potentially harmful bacteria.

Aluminum

Aluminum is a lightweight metal found naturally in large quantities in the environment. Found in:

- Vaccines
- Drinking water
- Metal pipes
- Ingesting foods
- Infant formula
- Pots and pans
- Beverage cans
- Roofing
- Foil
- Antacids
- Buffered aspirin
- Food additives
- Antiperspirants

Dangers - Strong healthy kidneys can rid their bodies of the majority of aluminum from vaccines. However, infants have reduced renal function at birth, which does not reach maturity until 1-2 years. Young babies may not be able to excrete the aluminum from their bodies. Based on the toxicity thresholds, a 6lb baby could not handle more than (.014mg) of aluminum. The Hepatitis B vaccine, which is given at birth, contains **(.25mg) which is 20x the toxicity threshold.** Aluminum toxicity causes - encephalitis, bone disease, anemia, and can cross the blood brain barrier. The American Academy of Pediatrics has stated that aluminum is now being implicated as interfering with a variety of cellular and metabolic processes in the nervous system and other tissue.

Aluminum is still found in 8 major vaccines; DTP, Haemophilus Influenzae, Pneumococcal, Hepatitis A, Hepatitis B, Human Papillomavirus, Anthrax, and Rabies vaccines. (Refer to the full disclosure of all vaccines containing aluminum at **http://www.cdc.gov/vaccines/pubs/pinkbook/downloads/appendices/B/excipient-table-2.pdf**)

Antibiotics

Antibiotics are another ingredient contained in most vaccines that are given to babies and children. The most common type used of antibiotic used is called Neomycin. The real problem with antibiotics is the overuse and abuse of them. Over time their bodies, and ours, become antibiotic or antimicrobial resistant.

Found in

- Vaccines
- Meats
- Eggs
- Cheese
- Milk
- Processed food
- Fast foods
- Docs give sick kids

(Refer to the list above for full disclosure of all vaccines containing antibiotics)

When kids get sick we take them to the doctor who prescribes yet, another antibiotic. The over prescribed antibiotics make their bodies become resistant to the particular strain of antibiotic and the treatment is ineffective, unable to fight the infection, fungi, bacteria or virus. This is common for many prescriptions; our bodies get used to the medications and we need more. We make an appointment and back to the doctor we go for a stronger antibiotic to fight the infection.

The Center for Disease Control (CDC) states the following about Antimicrobial (antibiotic) resistance. **"Antimicrobial resistance is one of our most serious health threats. Infections from resistant bacteria are now too common, and some pathogens have even become resistant to multiple types or classes of antibiotics (antimicrobials used to treat bacterial infections).** Antibiotic-resistant infections can also come from the food we eat. The germs that contaminate food can be resistant because of the use of antibiotics in people and in food from animals. We can prevent many of these infections by using antibiotics carefully, and keeping salmonella and other bacteria out of the food we eat."

Egg Embryo

Viruses are grown in egg embryos. The virus is injected inside of an egg embryo with a syringe to be used in the vaccine.

Eggs found in:

- Omelets
- Waffles
- French toast
- Pancakes
- Salad dressings
- Pastas
- Mayonnaise
- Jarred goods
- Sauces
- Ice creams
- Puddings
- Prepackaged foods
- Baked goods
- Cakes
- Brownies
- Breads
- Egg rolls
- Canned soups

It is recommended by the CDC that

"Asthmatic patients and others with egg allergies might be denied active immunization because of the risk of inducing adverse reactions with a vaccine derived from egg embryo tissue. If you are thinking about giving your child vaccines, make sure your child has had no reactions to eggs as a precaution. Parents should contact their doctors with their child's prior history of any allergic reactions to eggs."

Read the labels: under the names of globulin, lecithin, albumin, simplesse, lysozyme, ovalbumin, ovomucin, ovomucoid which still contain egg whites.

Most children that are allergic to eggs are reacting to the protein in the egg whites or the yoke; this usually shows up when children are very young. When you have an allergy to anything, your immune system overreacts to the protein in that food causing an allergic reaction.

Dangers: Egg Allergies

- Anaphylaxis
- Death
- Trouble breathing
- Wheezing
- Throat tightness
- Stomach aches
- Swelling
- Hives
- Diarrhea
- Vomiting
- Swollen eyes
- Drop in blood pressure

Emergencies

It may start with milder symptoms but can become worse very quickly. You will need to rush your child to an emergency hospital or call 911 for immediate assistance. If your child has an allergy to eggs, please take the proper precautions and never get a vaccine in a drugstore or supermarket.

Egg Embryos – used in flu vaccines. The measles and mumps viruses are grown on a culture which contains chick embryo cells (not on eggs). Always check with your doctor to find out which vaccines are grown in egg embryos. (Refer to the full disclosure of all vaccines containing Egg embryos, **http://www.cdc.gov/vaccines/pubs/pinkbook/downloads/appendices/B/excipient-table-2.pdf)**

Formaldehyde

Most of us do not know what formaldehyde is except that undertakers use it to preserve the body until the funeral takes place. Formaldehyde is a colorless gas with a rather strong odor; used to inactivate viruses so the child does not contract the disease associated in the vaccine.

Found In:

- Vaccines
- Textile industries
- Resins
- Adhesives
- Plywood
- Carpet
- Crease-resistant fabrics
- Facial tissues
- Paper towels
- Napkins
- Paints
- Foams
- Insulation

Our bodies also produce and use formaldehyde when we ingest foods like citric fruits and juices, vegetables, fermented beverages, plants, and animals. Our bodies use formaldehyde to form DNA and amino acids. However, we are injected with it and also eat and breathe it; it is in the napkins and facial tissues we use.

Dangers:

"Formaldehyde ingestion results in severe corrosive damage to the gastrointestinal tract followed by CNS depression, myocardial depression, circulatory collapse, metabolic acidosis and multiple organ failure. The toxic effects of formaldehyde in experimental animals include: irritation, cytotoxicity, and cell proliferation in the upper respiratory tract, ocular irritation, pulmonary hyperactivity, bronchoconstriction, gastrointestinal irritation, and skin sensitization. Other reported effects include oxidative stress, neurotoxicity, neurobehavioral effects, immunotoxicity, testicular toxicity, and decreased liver, thyroid gland, and testis weights." (IARC 2006, Asian et al. 2006, Sarsilmaz et al. 2007, Golalipour et al. 2008, Ozen et al. 2005, Majumder and Kumar 1995).

FDA states "Formaldehyde has induced a rare form of nasal cancer in both Fischer 344 rats and in B6C3F1 mice as reported in an ongoing study by the C I I T.

Formaldehyde found in vaccines: Hepatitis B vaccine (HBVaxPro), Preschool Booster vaccines (Repevax), Teenage Booster vaccine (Revaxis), (Polio virus vaccine) and (diphtheria vaccine.)

Mercury - Thimerosal

Mercuric chloride (HgCl2) is a very poisonous salt once used to disinfect wounds. Thimerosal is a poison, neurotoxin, cancer-causer, and can interrupt the immune system as well as the normal development of an unborn baby or a child. It has been widely used as a preservative in a number of drug products, including vaccines to help prevent potentially life threatening contamination with harmful microbes. Thimerosal is so toxic that putting it on your skin is illegal. However, mercury is added to the influenza vaccines which can be especially dangerous to pregnant women and newborn children.

Found In:

- Vaccines
- Fish
- Thermometers
- Barometers
- Streetlights
- Fluorescent Lights
- Advertising signs
- Dental amalgams (filings)
- Batteries
- Red paint

Mercury enters the body through the respiratory tract, the digestive tract or directly through the skin. It accumulates in the body eventually causing severe illness or death.

"The Food and Drug Administration has worked with vaccine manufacturers to reduce or eliminate thimerosal from vaccines. It has been removed from or reduced to trace amounts in all vaccines routinely recommended for children 6 years of age and younger, with the exception of inactivated influenza vaccine." Vaccines with trace amounts of thimerosal contain 1 microgram or less of mercury per dose.

Some research states that even trace amounts of mercury are still too much for an infant and should be eliminated completely.

To find out what Current chemical additives are in specific vaccines, ask your healthcare provider or pharmacist for a copy of the vaccine package insert, which lists all ingredients in the vaccine and discusses any known adverse reactions.

Dangers of Toxins in Vaccines, Foods & Products

Vaccinations are probably one of the most controversial topics investigated worldwide for children's health. I present the facts and the information from the FDA site including vaccine history, studies, and ingredients.

- They are injected into small babies where their immune system or the blood brain barrier has not developed fully yet.

- Toxins are brought into the body through injections, ingesting toxins through food and drinks, and breathing in toxins, making this a dangerous combination and accumulation of toxins into a very young baby.

- The FDA states vaccines are safe for healthy babies. However, I hypothesize that most babies are born unhealthy from living inside unhealthy mommies where toxins cross the placenta from mommy to baby.

- Our bodies make formaldehyde which is one of the ingredients in vaccines. If we produce formaldehyde, eat it, breathe it through paints, napkins and facial tissues, and are injected with the vaccine, are we overdosing on formaldehyde?

- Babies are raised with fast foods, pre-packaged foods, white flours and sugars loaded with dangerous and unhealthy ingredients. They are all packed into baby foods, table foods and formulas. If our babies are being dosed with toxins from all these sources: foods, the air we breathe, and products we use, could the dose from a vaccine be the missing link that is pushing our kids over the edge and contributing to the rise in diseases such as SIDS, Autism, ADD, and ADHD?

- There are extreme amounts of vaccines given to children before their first birthday. More than ten million vaccines are administered to children that are less than one year, and usually between 2 and 6 months.

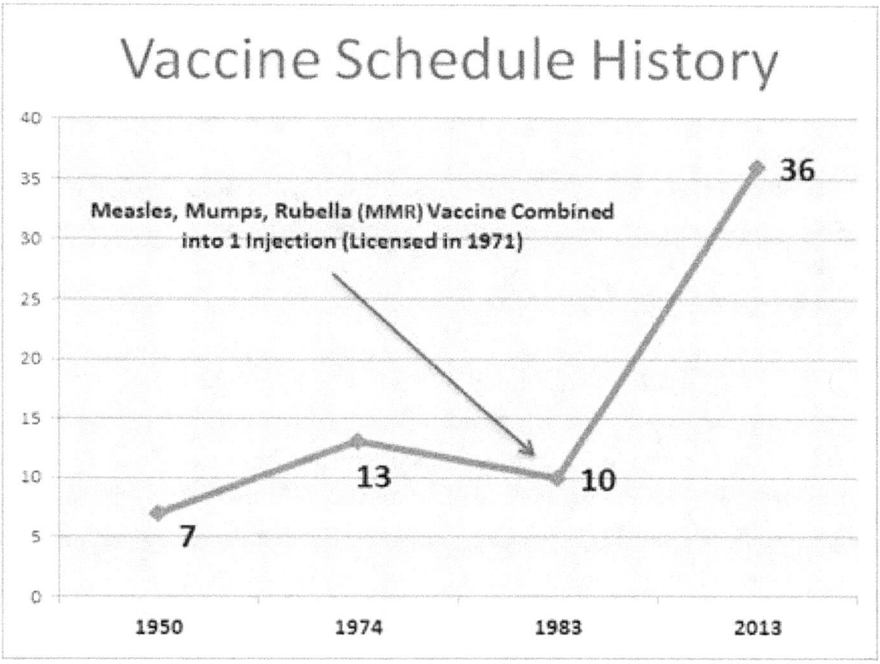

As you can see, children's vaccines have greatly increased from only seven in 1950 - 1970 to a whopping 36 in 2013. I grew up in the 1950's; all of my friends and I lived through having chicken pocks, mumps and measles. Today's researchers and doctors would rather you have a vaccine instead of actually getting the virus. Another school of thought invites you to a party; "a pox party", where parents bring their kids over so they can get a case of chickenpox. It is very contagious and children catch it though coughs and sneezes or touching the blisters. Pox parties, held in the 50's and today, are tailored for young children since it can be more serious for teens and adults. People feel their kids have stronger immune systems after having the virus. Doctors feel it is safer to be injected with the vaccine, even though vaccines carry other dangerous ingredients along with part of the virus.

Current Doses of Vaccines

49 Doses of 14 Vaccines Before Age 6

60 Doses of 16 Vaccines Before Age 18

What Causes Infections?

- Alcohol
- Smoking
- Antibiotics
- Overeating
- Toxic foods
- Stress
- Cooked foods
- Over exertion
- Medications
- Hormones
- Pesticides
- Not enough sleep

Types of Infection- When to Use Antibiotics

A letter published in the Journal of the American Medical Association shows "doctors prescribe antibiotics for acute bronchitis approximately 70% of the time, despite years of evidence demonstrating that these drugs do not work against respiratory illness. Viruses usually cause the common cold and influenza with upper respiratory infections, so antibiotic will not work". In fact, antibiotics will lower your immune system and upset your digestive tract, which is where 70 percent of your immune system is. Antibiotics work best for bacterial infections, not viruses. When you get viruses, they usually will just run their course. Taking immune boosters may be a better idea to help reduce the time you are ill. Always consult your doctor for medical advice. However, educate yourself and know the difference between bacterial and viral illnesses.

<u>Bacterial</u> – NEED ANTIBIOTICS - ear infections (caused by bacteria), stomach aches, chest or sinus infections, strep throat, bronchitis caused by bacteria, pink eye (bacteria), pneumonia

<u>Viruses</u> – DO NOT NEED ANTIBIOTICS - colds, flu, herpes, measles, bronchitis caused by virus, sore throat, upper respiratory infections, sinusitis, ear infection (caused by virus)

<u>Fungi</u> – thrush, athlete's foot

Prevention is Better than Cure

Antibiotics are necessary in acute situations and emergencies because they can save a life, but the CDC states they are over prescribed and over used.

Building our immune systems should be first and foremost in the steps we take to make and heal ourselves and our children.

Natural Alternatives - Immune Boosters

Herbs are medicinal plants (also called "phytomedicinals") that can be administered as the whole plant or plant parts or by extracting one or more ingredients using solvents to yield tinctures, tea or other extracts. Synthetic drugs (what the drug industry calls "pharmaceuticals") are synthesized chemically in the laboratory to produce drugs not found in nature. One quarter of the drugs used in the United States are derived from plants such as opiates, digitalis, and Taxol. The active ingredient(s) are extracted from the plant, replicating it's structure in the lab then mass producing it. Herbal drugs are considered less potent than prescribed medicines. The latter usually contains one highly concentrated active ingredient, while herbs may have several active ingredients that are chemically similar. Herbal ingredients work synergistically to contribute to, or detract from, the therapeutic effect of each individual ingredient.

The following are recommended supplements that help to boost the immune system and fight off infections. You can look for these ingredients in your local health food store. You can also eat your way to good health by incorporating antioxidants to detoxify the body by using vitamins A, C, E, beta-carotene, zinc, selenium Co-Q-lO, DHA, and EFA into your diet. You can get natural beta-carotene by eating fresh red, orange and yellow vegetables like red watermelon, colored peppers, orange carrots and cantaloupe.

Echinacea - antiviral and antibacterial properties
Garlic - contains allicin, antiviral, antifungal and antibacterial
Ginger great for sore throat and upset stomachs
Goldenseal - natural antibacterial, good for digestive health
Grapefruit Seed Extract - powerful antibiotic, antifungal and antiviral agent
Mushrooms - shiitake, maitake, reishi or ganodenna (great for liver health)

Probiotics alternative to antibiotics, provide beneficial bacteria to the digestive track instead of robbing it

Recommended Immune Boosters and Infection Fighters from Premier Research Labs

Allicidin

Live-Source Stabilized Garlic Extracts For Powerful Immune Regulation

Premier Allicidin™ features allicin, the most powerful compound found in garlic and European wild garlic, called Bear's Garlic, the original non-hybrid garlic (not common kitchen garlic). It is antibacterial, antifungal, anti-parasitic and antiviral.

Nucleo Immune

Research shows that nucleotides can help the body to rapidly overcome colds or flu, heal wounds, improve circulation, strengthen the immune system, promote new cell growth, neutralize toxins (especially in the intestines), enhance the body's ability to fight infection and disease, and may even help slow the aging process.

HCL

Premier Betaine HCL is created to assist the body's natural stomach acids in digestion and absorption of nutrients, especially protein, vitamin B12, calcium, iron and other minerals. Healthy stomach acid is needed for a healthy digestive tract. With low stomach acid, even the best food cannot be properly digested. The inability to absorb nutrients properly can lead to serious health problems. Healthy stomach acid helps kill disease-causing microbes and parasites routinely found in food. With low stomach acid, these infecting invaders may not be destroyed by the stomach's acid bath therefore potentially causing many types of infections. This is why low stomach acid (hypochlorhydria) is associated with so many common health problems.

Probiotic Caps

Powerful, broad-spectrum "good bacteria" for ideal intestinal ecology

- 59,000,000 CFU lactic acid bacteria per capsule
- Contains more than 12 different strains of beneficial probiotic bacteria
- Unique Japanese process using 92 different natural herbs and barks, cultured for 5 years
- Ideal for everyone, including infants
- Highly biologically available source of 10 vitamins, 8 minerals and 18 amino acids
- Certified as 6.25 times stronger than any other lactic acid bacteria
- 3-year shelf life
- Fully "live" raw nutrient concentrate; not freeze-dried
- One of the finest products for beneficial bacterial re-inoculation
- Suppresses the growth of harmful micro-organisms
- Supports regular bowel movements; helps the body overcome diarrhea (often infection-based)
- Delivers significant amounts of four organic acids critical to enzyme synthesis

Olive Leaf Supports

Comprehensive blend of nutrients to support the immune system. Specifically good for antiviral activity support

- Weakened Immune System
- Giardia, Chlamydia, Clostridium, Helicobacter
- Osteoarthritis and Rheumatoid Arthritis
- Healthy Blood Pressure
- Arrhythmias
- Fungus Infections (jock itch, athletes foot, fungal nails, etc.).

- Viral Infections (herpes, influenza, colds, cytomegalovirus, Epstein-Barr virus, retroviruses)

Oregano Oil

The most active ingredient in wild oregano is carvacrol, a potent naturally occurring compound which has remarkable effects to support and promote the immune system; an excellent antioxidant. It takes 100 pounds of oregano plants to make 1 pound of the essential oil of oregano. This concentrated natural oil is very powerful. Premier Oregano Oil contains over 50 compounds, which possess immune promoting actions.

- Broad-spectrum immune support
- Concentrated genuine oil of oregano; naturally contains over 50 powerful, immune-specific compounds
- Always keep a bottle on hand, ready for any acute problem (such as onset of colds, flu or respiratory disturbances)
- Also helps with nausea & food poisoning

Mix 2 drops Premier Oregano Oil with 2 drops Limonene in water. Gargle and swallow every few hours or as often as necessary.

Premier Oregano Oil is the essential oil of oregano, specifically Origanum vulgare which is the true, oregano species. Unbelievably, most oregano and oregano oils available in the U.S. are from non-oregano species, primarily marjoram or thyme, and they are actually falsely labeled!

Aloe Mannan-FX

Advanced immune and gastrointestinal support with volcanic grown aloe

- Immune system prevention and recovery support
- Immuno-stimulant, antiviral, antineoplastic and properties
- May reduce mycotoxic body burden, especially in sinuses
- Guaranteed minimum of 1/8 tsp. of acemannan

- Uniquely fermented with patented calcium bentonite and Luo Han Guo extract for added support

Aloe Mannan-FX is derived from Aloe barbadensis, rich in the key compound, acemannan. This extraordinary, one-of-a-kind aloe is meticulously grown in open sea air on a volcanic island in rich volcanic soil.

Raintree Supplement

Cats Claw

Very powerful antiviral, antioxidant and immune boosting agent (recommend online purchasing from **Raintree Formula**)

http://www.raintree.com/cats-claw-capsules?gclid=CjwKEAjwya-6BRDR3p6FuY2-u3MSJAD1paxTzAAVo7Z1UPF2Zjz5BtJDxGuykRZa-reaU-Ult5mJcrhoCdy7w_wcB

Children at Risk – Vaccines, Government & Big Pharma's Dirty Money

Robert F. Kennedy, Jr. is stated as saying, "...that every vaccine introduced to the vaccine schedule guarantees its manufacturer millions of customers, increasing vaccine revenue by billions of dollars. However, it appears that a minimum of 56 doses of 14 vaccinations before the age of eighteen is not quite lucrative enough for the pharmaceutical industry", as according to Mr. Kennedy's research, "the CDC has 271 new vaccinations under development in the hopes that vaccine revenues will reach a staggering $100 billion by 2025". Kennedy called the Centers for Disease Control and Prevention (CDC) "a cesspool of corruption, mismanagement and dysfunction, making it crystal clear to readers that financial gain fueled their decision making.""

Dr. Martin Luther King, Jr. "Of all the forms of inequality, injustice in health care is the most shocking and inhumane."

Dangers with the Flu Vaccine

This is a copy of the Flulaval (Influenza Virus Vaccine) for 2013 -2014. There are concerns for safety for young children, pregnant or nursing mothers.

FLULAVAL® (Influenza Virus Vaccine)
Suspension for Intramuscular Injection
2013-2014 Formula

8.3 Nursing Mothers

It is not known whether FLULAVAL is excreted in human milk. Because many drugs are excreted in human milk, caution should be exercised when FLULAVAL is administered to a nursing woman.

8.4 Pediatric Use

Safety and effectiveness of FLULAVAL in pediatric patients have not been established.

8.5 Geriatric Use

In clinical trials, there were 330 subjects who were ≥65 years of age and received FLULAVAL; 142 of these subjects were ≥75 years of age. Hemagglutination-inhibiting (HI) antibody responses were lower in geriatric subjects than younger subjects after administration of FLULAVAL. *[See Clinical Studies (14.2).]* Solicited adverse events were similar in frequency to those reported in younger subjects *[see Adverse Reactions (6.1)]*.

11 DESCRIPTION

FLULAVAL, Influenza Virus Vaccine, for intramuscular injection, is a trivalent, split-virion, inactivated influenza virus vaccine prepared from virus propagated in the allantoic cavity of embryonated hens' eggs. Each of the influenza virus strains is produced and purified separately. The virus is inactivated with ultraviolet light treatment followed by formaldehyde treatment, purified by centrifugation, and disrupted with sodium deoxycholate.

FLULAVAL is a sterile, translucent to whitish opalescent suspension in a phosphate-buffered saline solution that may sediment slightly. The sediment resuspends upon shaking to form a homogeneous suspension. FLULAVAL has been standardized according to USPHS requirements for the 2013-2014 influenza season and is formulated to contain 45 mcg hemagglutinin (HA) per 0.5-mL dose in the recommended ratio of 15 mcg HA of each of the following 3 strains: A/California/7/2009 NYMC X-179A (H1N1), A/Texas/50/2012 NYMC X-223A (H3N2) (an A/Victoria/361/2011-like virus), and B/Massachusetts/2/2012 NYMC BX-51B.

Thimerosal, a mercury derivative, is added as a preservative. Each 0.5-mL dose contains 50 mcg thimerosal (<25 mcg mercury). Each 0.5-mL dose may also contain residual amounts of ovalbumin (≤0.3 mcg), formaldehyde (≤25 mcg), and sodium deoxycholate (≤50 mcg) from the manufacturing process. Antibiotics are not used in the manufacture of this vaccine.

The vial stoppers are not made with natural rubber latex.

12 CLINICAL PHARMACOLOGY

12.1 Mechanism of Action

Influenza illness and its complications follow infection with influenza viruses. Global surveillance of influenza identifies yearly antigenic variants. For example, since 1977, antigenic variants of influenza A (H1N1 and H3N2) viruses and influenza B viruses have been in global circulation. Specific levels of HI antibody titer post-vaccination with inactivated influenza virus vaccines have not been correlated with protection from influenza illness but the antibody titers have been used as a measure of vaccine activity. In some human challenge studies, antibody titers of ≥1:40 have been associated with protection from influenza illness in up to 50% of subjects.[1,2] Antibody against one influenza virus type or subtype confers little or no protection against another virus. Furthermore, antibody to one antigenic variant of influenza virus might not protect against a new antigenic variant of the same type or subtype. Frequent development of antigenic variants through antigenic drift is the virological basis for seasonal epidemics and the reason for the usual change of one or more new strains in each year's influenza vaccine. Therefore, inactivated influenza vaccines are standardized to contain the hemagglutinins of strains (i.e., typically 2 type A and 1 type B), representing the influenza viruses likely to circulate in the United States in the upcoming winter.

Annual revaccination with the current vaccine is recommended because immunity declines during the year after vaccination, and because circulating strains of influenza virus change from year to year.[3]

13 NONCLINICAL TOXICOLOGY

13.1 Carcinogenesis, Mutagenesis, Impairment of Fertility

FLULAVAL has not been evaluated for carcinogenic or mutagenic potential, or for impairment of fertility.

The following is a comparison for the vaccination Instructions that come with the vaccine from 2013-2014 to the last revised in June of 2015.

1. Nursing Mothers: It is not known if Flulaval is excreted in human milk when breastfeeding and caution should be exercised. This is still the same. **Since they are not sure if the ingredients pass from mother to child during breastfeeding, it may be advisable not to get any flu vaccines while you are breastfeeding.**

2. Pediatric Use: Safety and effectiveness in pediatric patients has not been evaluated. New 2015 states the safety and effectiveness in children below the age of 6 months have not been evaluated**. Is it worth the gamble to have a vaccine or the flu shot Fluvanal, administered to any child under the age of 6 months since the safety has not been evaluated?**

3. Description: This 2013-2014 copy of the vaccine Flulaval shows the use of Thimerosal, a mercury derivative as an added preservative. However, in the 2015 copy it has been removed from the single dose but is still listed and contained in the 5ml multi dose vaccine showing: Thimerosal, a mercury derivative contains 25 mcg mercury. **If you decide to use a flu shot for your child, at the very least administer to a child over the age of 6 months and only use the single dose vaccine without the use of Thimerosal. Remember there are still reported trace amounts of mercury used.**

4. Nonclinical Toxicology: The 2013-2014 copy notes that it has not been evaluated for carcinogenic (cancer causing), mutagenic (a change to genetic material that may cause cancer) or impairment of fertility (unable to become pregnant). However, in the 2015 copy, section 13 has been completely eliminated; the new copy jumps from number 12 to 14. **This seems odd that this section was taken out without even changing the numbers.**

8

"HONEY, I BLEW UP THE KIDS" FAT KIDS & DIABETES

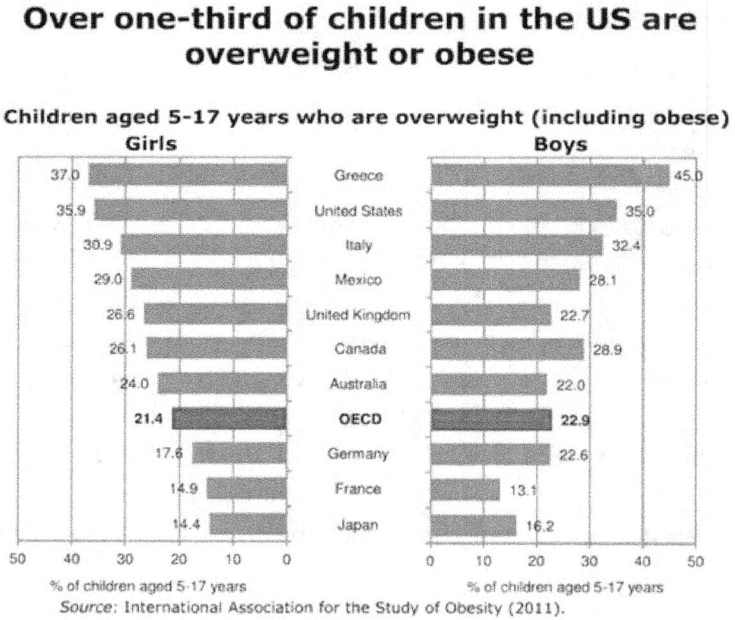

Prevalence of Childhood Obesity in the United States, 2011-2012

Childhood obesity is a serious problem in the United States. For children and adolescents aged 2-19 years, the prevalence of obesity has remained fairly stable at about 17% and affects about 12.7 million children and adolescents for the past decade.

Our Kids Getting Geriatric Diseases

- About 208,000 Americans under age 20 are estimated to have diagnosed diabetes, approximately 0.25% of that population. (American Diabetes Association)
- Type 2 diabetes develops most often in middle-aged and older adults but is now becoming more common in our children.
- For more information, visit: http://www.diabetes.org/diabetes-basics/statistics/?referrer=https://www.google.com/#sthash.fEzf7Z9P.dpuf

"Eat McDonalds and Become a Big Mac"

- One in four people in America visit a fast food restaurant every day
- Fast food restaurants distribute many toys to children
- Contribute to obesity and disease
- Approximately 50 million people eat at McDonald's everyday

High Calories in Fast Food Restaurants

- White Castle - 20 chicken rings = 1,760 calories
- Burger King - Ultimate breakfast platter = 1,450 calories
- McDonald's - Big breakfast w/ syrup and margarine = 1,350 calories
- KFC - 10-piece original recipe chicken bites = 1,300 calories
- Wendy's - Hot 'N Juicy 3/4 lb. triple w/ cheese = 1,120 calories
- Panera Bread - Steak and white cheddar on baguette = 980 calories
- Taco Bell - Volcanic nachos = 970 calories
- Dunkin' Donuts - Frozen mocha coffee coolatta = 730 calories
- Subway - Mega melt on flatbread with egg = 660 calories
- Pizza Hut - 14-inch large meat lover's pan pizza = 470 calories per slice
- Burger King Triple Whopper = 1,020 calories
- Quizno's large Veggie Deluxe sandwich = 1,060 calories
- Cinnabon's Caramel Pecanbon = 1,080 calories
- Mountain Dew Baja Blast at Taco Bell XL = 1,134 calories

"Holy Kleenex Batman, it was right under our noses and we blew it! – Robin!"

You blew it all right, if you continue on the fast food track. Just looking at the above calories should be a major deterrent to never go to a fast food restaurant. Moreover, if you think you can get away with just a drink, check out the whopping calorie drinks at Dunkin Donuts and Taco Bell. Do not be fooled, there are hidden calories and junk at almost all fast food restaurants. Fast food can increase the risk of hardening and narrowing of the arteries, heart disease and stroke due to the types of ingredients it contains and the high quantities that people consume.

Let's talk junk in fast food

Trans fats - saturated trans fats add hydrogen to liquid vegetable oils. Trans fats, also known as partially hydrogenated oils, raise your unhealthy cholesterol levels, leading to fatty plaques and hardening of the arteries.

Sugar - is included in all beverages such as fruit juice, milkshakes, and sodas. High sugar consumption can lead to obesity and an increase in Type 2 diabetes.

Sodium – Commercial processing and preparation make fast foods high in sodium. French Fries add 335mg before they have been sprinkled with salt, two pancakes with syrup have 1,104mg of sodium, and a roast beef sandwich contains 792mg of sodium. The average consumption of sodium for a healthy person is 2300mg. I recommend using pink salt from Premier and do not consume the unhealthy white salt used in most restaurants.

Calories - Weight gain and obesity. When eating at a fast food restaurant we usually eat too many calories all at one time. High fat and sugar content can lead to cardiovascular disease.

Chipotle is a recommended fast food restaurant due to their large choice of organic and responsibly raised products. To make it healthy, order a salad with organic beans. If you pass on the cheese you can keep it healthy and lower in calories. Even though their cheese is actually organic, I am not a fan of cheese products for anyone.

"Play Ball"

Strike one – You have one overweight parent. I am not talking about overweight parents as adults because half the population is there. I am talking about large as a child. My dad was also large as a child and had to wear husky clothes; so was I.

Strike two – You are female. Women have a higher percentage of body fat than men. Men have more muscle making their metabolism more efficient. Muscle burns more fat even while a person is at their resting metabolic rate.

Strike three - You are feeding your children carbs (flour products, fast food, processed foods, sugar)

You are not out.... you just need to keep your eye on the ball.

"Fat is as Fat Does" Fat Kids Beware

Everyone is born with a certain number of fat cells. As an adult we can have between 10 and 30 billion fat cells. So if we pig out and gain weight when we are young, the fat cells start adding up, increasing the amount of fat cells. So a young person or child that is overweight as a child will have more fat cells than someone that was not overweight, usually twice the amount. The good news is you can lose them while you are still a child. Unfortunately, by the time we reach 20 we cannot lose fat cells, so you are stuck with the increased amount.

But get this...you can still increase the amount of fat cells; the more you eat and gain, those fat cells keep expanding and if they get big enough they start to divide and create more cells. Well that's not fair! Then as we age our fat cells start to die off, well that sounds good, right? No, as they die off they regenerate, keeping that dreaded number of fat cells the same. The more fat cells we have, the harder it is to lose weight. It's ok...we can still lose weight by reducing the amount of fat in the cell, making us a mean, lean machine! It may be too late for us to reduce the amount of fat cells, but if you have small children, make sure they do not become overweight during childhood.

Another problem is many of us that are dieting do not include good fats. Our bodies need healthy fat to burn fat. If we do not get enough fat, we turn into little gremlins, screaming "FEED ME." If you don't add in some good fat, what do you think you will start to crave? FAT and most likely the wrong kind, like french fries and chicken.

Research shows our genes can't be changed, but they can be turned on with exercise. If you are the kind of person that eats a donut and it goes right to your butt, then exercise is now your new best friend. The phenomenon is called epigenetics, DNA methylation. DNA is in every cell and has our own little blueprint of who we are and who are parents were. So guess what? Exercise puts your gene in overdrive....it revs up those fat genes.

"Exercise, You Don't Have Time Not To"

Read "Let's Go Out to the Ball Game" on Exercise Chapter 4 ADHD

New research from Lund University in Sweden, reported in PLoS Genetics June 27, 2013, described for the first time what happens in fat cells when we exercise. They studied the methyl groups in fat cells of 23 overweight and inactive men around 35 years old. These men exercised twice a week for six months doing either a spin class or aerobics class. What they found was that exercise altered the methylation pattern in 7,000 out of 480,000 genes that were observed. **It changed the pattern of fat storage in the genes.** Another study compared the gene alteration from a group that burned off 400 calories. One group burned it with an intense workout, the other group with a low impact workout. What they found was intensity does matter. The group that worked out harder had more change to the fat in their gene storage. It also showed that just one workout can also affect your gene mutation.

"Thing 1, Thing 2"

There have been many studies done with twins that support the genetic weight factor. James C. Romeis, a professor of health services researcher and investigator stated that "About 50 percent of adult-onset weight change remains genetic." He studied almost 4,000 sets of male twins who served in the military during the Vietnam War. The study revealed that genes account for 50 percent of the change in body mass index and the other 50 percent is due to diet and exercise.

Remy Cooks Up a Mutated Gene – The Mrap2 gene

In the Journal of Science and the Journal of Clinical Investigation, researchers describe new genetic factors that help to describe weight gain in people. Researchers at the Boston Children's Hospital found a rare genetic mutation that prevented mice from burning off fat calories. The mutation, Mrap2gene, showed that they fed a group of mice with this mutated gene less food and they still gained weight. When they fed the mice the same amount of calories as the group with no mutation, they noticed the mice continued to gain weight. The control group did not gain weight like the mutated mice. They also found the **same gene was mutated in a group of obese people.** The studies found that weight gain is a combination of different metabolic processes, from brain systems that regulate appetite to enzymes that control how calories are turned from food into either energy or fat. The scientists found a similar pattern among a group of 500 obese people; they detected four mutations in the human version of Mrap2, and each of the obese individuals possessed only one bad version of the gene.

9

"TWINKLE TWINKLE" - TOO MUCH TECHNOLOGY

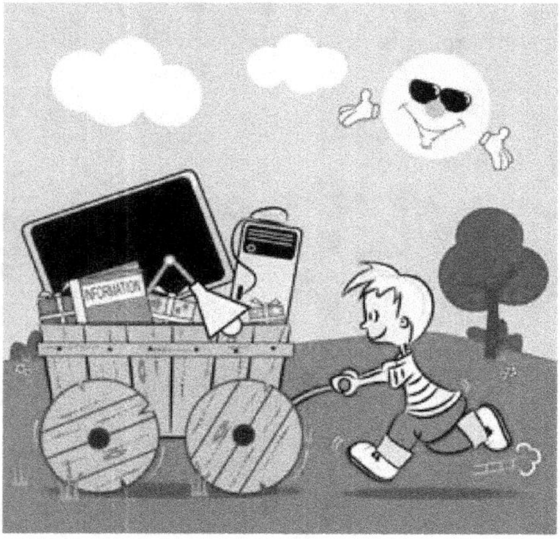

Technology or better named the "bad babysitter", includes the games and movies on our phones, computers and iPads that have replaced human interactions. Just like the carb/sugar addiction, the technology is also an addiction. Why do you think our kids want more and more, holler, and cry when we take them away? Many parents are tired, patience is short and we reach for the iPad to sooth our cranky babies and to give us a break. Parents cannot compete with the colorful 3D graphics and exquisitely choreographed movies and games that suck our children in. Have you ever wondered what effect the Electro Magnet Field (EMF) pollution is doing to our children's bodies at such an early age? We will explore the physical, mental and emotional effects this excessive energy has on their bodies through proven scientific studies.

Electromagnetic (EM) radiation is transmitted in waves or particles at different wavelengths and frequencies. This broad range of wavelengths is known as the electromagnetic spectrum. EM is defined as, "Radiation involves a transfer of energy through space. Depending on the amount of energy carried by radiation, radiation can be classified into ionizing radiation and nonionizing radiation. The main difference between ionizing and nonionizing radiation is that ionizing radiation refers to types of radiation where the radiation carries enough energy to ionize atoms, whereas nonionizing radiation refers to types of radiation that do not carry enough energy to ionize atoms".

The four forms of electromagnetic radiation include

1. **Electric** - Anything with an electric field flowing through it including the power l   ines that transport it

Lower frequency sources:

- High and low voltage electric power lines
- Solar panels
- Electric substations
- Street power converters
- Electric transportation power lines

Higher frequency sources:

- Wireless communication facilities
- Cell phone tower
- TV and radio broadcasting stations
- Wi-Fi and Wi-Max regional communication equipment
- "Smart City" components
- Military communications, radar and electronic warfare equipment

2. **Magnetic** - Anything having a magnetic field, which could come from an electric source or from a motor or engine
✥ Stainless steel (SS) cookware ✥ SS utensils ✥ SS sink ✥ SS scouring sponge (surprise!) ✥ Mandolin ✥ Washing machine drum ✥ Fridge casing ✥ Eyelash curler ✥ Tweezer ✥ Scissors, plier, shears, can-opener and knife ✥ Cast iron cookware ✥ Cast iron stove cap and grid

✣ Baking tray ✣ Nickel jewelry ✣ Jar lid ✣ Food can ✣ Tea/cookie tin ✣ Paint can ✣ Sewing needle ✣ Hammer, wrench and spanner ✣ Allen key ✣ Screwdriver head ✣ Bolt and nut ✣ Concrete nail ✣ Wood nail ✣ Screw and screw hook ✣ Spring ✣ Picture hanging plate ✣ Keyring ✣ Paper clip ✣ Binder clip ✣ Round binder clip ✣ Staple ✣ Steel rule ✣ Safety pin ✣ Watch battery ✣ Batteries, such as AA and AAA ✣ USB drive connector

3. **Wireless/RF** - Anything that communicates with a wireless signal using
   a. radio frequency
   b. microwave
   c. Wi-Fi - thermostats, cameras, remote car starters, cell phones, refrigerators iPods, iPads, computers, routers, televisions with satellite connections

4. **Ionizing** - Includes gamma rays, Ultraviolet rays, tanning booth, and X-rays.

Gamma rays have the smallest wavelengths and the most energy of any wave in the electromagnetic spectrum. The hottest and most energetic objects in the universe produce them. They are also used to treat cancer.

Very young kids are starting their educational life with the latest and greatest technology with iPads, smart phones and computers. My grandson Casher, is not even two years old and knows all his colors, 1-10 numbers and the alphabet, which is very common today. However, Casher has learned most of his information with old-fashioned books, puzzles, flash cards and of course some from computer programs and television.

"The Choice of a New Generation"

"Beauty or the Beast", When is technology too much? For many kids today, technology is both the teacher and babysitter. What happens when you take the babysitter away? Does your little beauty turn into a beast? I see it everywhere

I go…restaurants, grocery stores and even at family gatherings. Ok I get it! I know being a working parent is difficult; work, dinner, kid time, spouse time and then the cranky time. It works! Babies and kids get cranky and you wave your magic wand and presto, no more cranky!

It is becoming the norm to see our toddlers and school-aged children playing games, doing homework and they make navigating the internet look easy. In fact, they end up showing their parents things. We have to accept that the iPhone and iPad are the future and are here to stay. Kids will need to be skilled in technology since they are used in schools and especially for the future jobs markets. A child that is limited to technology and does not have a parent working at home with them, will most likely not be as educated as someone with technology is.

Kids love the bright colors, the challenge, and the sound effects to pull them in. The downfall of this buzz is that children using too much technology have been known to:

1. Become lazy
2. Do not learn good communication skills
3. Become addicted and dependent
4. Become depressed and anxious
5. Need instant gratification and be distracted
6. Have physical problems with their neck and back
7. Have problems with eyes and children's brains

Dr. Doo Little – Lazy Kids

"According to a recent Ofcom report, 4 in 10 three and four-year-olds have access to a tablet at home and more than a third of children between the age of five and 15 have one of their own. We have seen a huge increase in the number of children presenting symptoms that relate to a sedentary life, particularly from age 11 onwards. This lifestyle is certainly contributing to childhood obesity and diabetes. Children of today do not have the muscle development since they are not outside playing games, riding bikes and participating in sports like the kids of yesteryears who were "stronger than dirt."

"Kids are so wired and tired they become lazy and crazy"

Research shows that time outdoors, especially interacting with nature, can restore attention, lower stress, and reduce aggression. It is so important to introduce your kids to the green grass and blue skies to help them grow healthier. They can get exposure to natural sunlight, play and interact with other kids, and exercise their bodies building stronger muscles and developing lasting relationships with friends. Kids experience natural increases in dopamine and serotonin by exercising which reduces anxiety, stress and anger. (Solutions in Chapter 4 ADHD/ADD under exercise)

"Live in Your World, Play in Ours" – Communicating & Making Friends

Living inside a computer game or movie seems to be more popular than playing in the great outdoors. It becomes easier to live inside our head. When we plug in we zone out and lose touch with the outside world! We sit alone, do not talk to anyone, stare at our computer screen, get distracted and engaged in games for hours. Our computers become our friends; they are easier, they do not fight back, call us names or beat us up. However, they also do not give us the opportunity to build a relationship or make a special friend to build a fort with, play baseball with, splash in a pool, play on a playground, spend the night and stay up late; we miss out on laughing, sharing private secrets and just being kids. The earlier a child interacts with other children, the easier it will be to interact with adults and others when they are older.

Let us not forget that good communication skills start as early as infancy. These learned skills help us solve problems, listen to others, express ourselves successfully, and form and maintain good interpersonal relationships. Mommies and daddies need to pay close attention to their kids and help them get through troubling times that crop up in many situations, especially with friends. It is up to us to teach our kids how to express what they are feeling in a comfortable way without feeling vulnerable, shy, afraid or intimidated. I know we all want our kids to make friends easily and be popular. There is nothing worse than when our kids come home and tell us that the kids at school would not play with them, made fun of or bullied them. It is important to teach our kids good self-esteem; keep open communication and help them learn how to express what they think and feel in a safe and comfortable way. Here are a few helpful communication skills to work on with your kids:

1. Teach them to listen to others – no one wants to be around someone that continuously talks creating a one sided relationship. This becomes boring and your child will have limited friends.
2. Teach your child to speak clearly so kids understand them
3. Teach your child not to insult others and to be compassionate and sensitive to the feelings of others.
4. Teach your child to make jokes, be light, funny, silly
5. Teach your child to stand up for themselves and not allow them to be pushed around.
6. Create fun into your kids' lives with special events and sleepovers with friends.

"They Can't Leave Home Without it" Addicted & Dependent

1. Do your kids constantly CRAVE the iPod? At the store, in the car, with dinner, in the restaurant, in front of TV, when getting dressed, at sports events?
2. Do they experience PLEASURE, become happier when you give it to them?
3. Do they have a LOSS OF CONTROL - cry, scream, kick, become physical, get depressed when you take it away?
4. Do they LACK MOTIVATION to do chores, exercise, and schoolwork?
5. Do they want MORE AND MORE time, more advanced games?

5 Stages of Addiction

1. Involves craving (want it all the time)
2. Pleasure when using (happy, laughing when gaming)
3. Loss of control over its use (need it, cry and scream when taken away)
4. Continued involvement despite adverse consequences (lack of motivation, mood changes)
5. Tolerance (need more and more of a drug)

If it walks like a duck and quacks like a duck......it must be a duck. Has your swan turned into an ugly duckling? If so, your first step with addiction is to admit your child has an addiction. This first step is sometimes the hardest because we actually have to admit to ourselves that we are somewhat responsible for letting this happen. We feel guilty. With any addiction, cold turkey will cause the entire family to suffer. When the addiction is taken away, there must always be a substitute to takes its place. After an alcoholic gives up alcohol, many substitute sugar products to curb their cravings. With a technology addiction, you will need to find substitutes that will help them to cope with their loss. Of course, an alcoholic will need to stay sober and not use at all. With technology, it will be a little different since you will just be limiting the computer usage.

"Life in the Fast Lane, Surely Makes You Lose Your Mind"

The "feel good" pleasure center turns on when they plug in. They get a high with watching a movie, playing a game, getting an email, tweet, or text. They feel connected and feel they have many friends (fake friends) through Facebook or text messages. The lights, sounds, actions, and violence feed their stress center or produces nor-epinephrine. Also, the need to go faster and faster produces a rush or high that makes them feel good.

It would be best to start on a weekend where you can devote time to helping your child transition. Check out the weather and pick a weekend where the weather is good. Depending on the severity of their addiction, your child may not be used to doing things on their own. You may become their new best friend. If they do not have many friends, you will need to find kids their age to interact with. Be patient with your child. This is a great chance to re-connect and improve your relationship with your children.

Here is a great book of activities to help get your kids to "back away from the iPod."

101 Kids Activities That Are the Bestest, Funnest Ever!: The Entertainment Solution for Parents, Relatives & Babysitters! Whether your kid is 3, 5 or 12 years old, there are hundreds of fun, educational and engaging things to do in this book. When they ask to watch television, you will have the perfect solution. *101 Kids Activities That Are the Bestest, Funnest Ever!* The book has time-tested, exciting activities to keep your children laughing and learning for the whole day, every day. Holly Homer and Rachel Miller are the women behind the wildly popular site *KidsActivitiesBlog.com*, which gets more than 2 million hits a month and has more than 71,000 fans on Facebook and 100,000 followers on Pinterest."

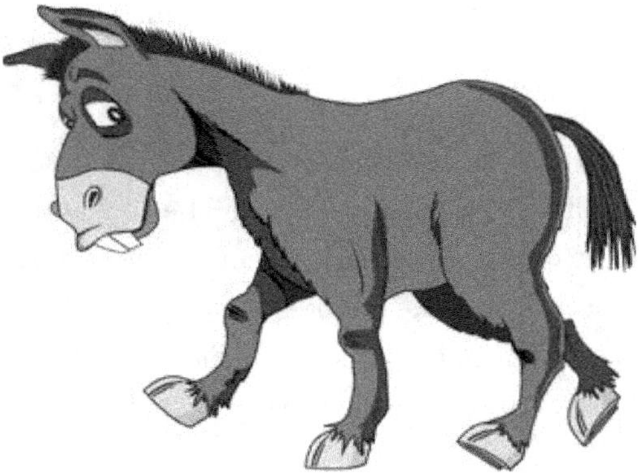

Eeyore says…
"It's not much of a tail, but I'm sort of attached to it." Depression & Anxiety
Computers can do more damage to mental health than good.

1. Much of the depression and anxiety is due to sleeping problems where kids have a hard time shutting down. The screens have intense lighting and colors, which keep them up even after the computer shuts down.
2. The second problem is lack of sunlight and exercise, which produces the "feel good" neurotransmitters dopamine and serotonin to keep us happy.
3. The third is feeling so high with the technology but without it they feel depressed.
4. The fourth is not developing communication skills and having a hard time in school making friends. This leads for feeling inferior to others and to having low self-esteem.

"Fast & Furious"

If you blink, you will miss him. He is the 10-year-old superhero, speedster Dash from The Incredibles. He is impulsive and reckless but he has a super suit that protects him from the wear and tear of his mistakes. However, our kids are vulnerable, so we must be that protective suit. We are super parents with cosmic powers sent here to defeat their weapons of destruction, their poisonous radiation, their kryptonite!

All you have to do is walk through a mall in your hometown and you will see people of all ages, but especially kids, looking down at their phones, anxiously awaiting their next response to a text or a like from Facebook or Instagram. Its kids on crack. phones always on, always connected, always wanting more and expecting it fast. Besides fast phones there are fast foods, fast cars, fast guitar players, fast rappers, fast internet connections, fast drugs (speed), and fast movies (on demand); we cook it fast, eat it fast, drink it fast. We are consumed with FAST...FAST...FAST! You can even get fast answers on *Google* to any question you can possibly think up. Your fingers no longer need to do the "walking through the yellow pages" when with the touch of a button or the sound of your voice you can find your way to your destination or to your favorite restaurant.

"Let 'er Rip Mr. Spacely"

Let us not forget the "far out", outer space 60's show *The Jetsons*, where their futuristic inventions have become a reality. We can rock it with flying cars (2017), jet packs, robotic house cleaners, drones, smart watches, video computers, dog treadmills, talking alarm clocks, and flat screen televisions. Most of us have to admit, we enjoy having computers that vacuum our homes, turns on our lights, enables us to see who is at the door when we are not home, talks to friends on watch phones, and protects our family from intruders. Computers are a way of life. However, it has created a "need for speed", and when we "don't have it our way" we become angry, impatient and frustrated. Waiting for anything produces anxiety and stress and many express their frustrations out on whomever they are closest to.

"Tech Neck" – Is your Neck in a Knot?

Giraffes are graceful, have a slow walk with their long neck swaying above the treetops always gazing and stretching their necks upward. Our kids are just the opposite. They are always looking down at their phones or posturing a stiff body while gaming. So is it no wonder that kids today are plagued with neck and back pain? They sit too long without stretching their bodies out. Kids also seem to be more hunched over when they walk which puts pressure and tension to the back, shoulders and neck. The solution to this is easy; make your kids go out and play in the dirt. Move it or lose it. For immediate relief from pain, a visit to your family chiropractor or massage therapist may be in order. Chiropractors will be able to correct the subluxation (a slight misalignment of the vertebrae, regarded in chiropractic theory as the cause of many health problems), and a massage therapist will be able to release muscle tension causing the pain. The two are like "two peas in a pod" and work very well together.

"See What We Think" Eyes and Brains

"Our eyes are the windows to our souls". We open them wide to see the beauty all around us. Today we seem to be in too much of a hurry to stop and "smell the roses." We miss an array of rainbow colors from glorious crimson sunsets, blue skies, green grasses and flowers of every color imaginable. We use our eyes for everything, but were they really meant to be used to stare at bright lights on a computer screen? We all turn on the bright lights everyday as we read on Kindles, use our smart phones, work and play on our laptops.

Some eye complaints people report are dry eyes, blurry eyes, and headaches. According to Dr. Richard Shugarman, a volunteer professor of ophthalmology at the Bascom Palmer Eye Institute at the University of Miami, "extremely high contrast from lit screens can cause headaches. Reading dark print on an extremely bright background can lead to spasms of the muscles at the temples, which causes stress headaches". Shugarman also believes that the blink rate slows down when you look at things up close, meaning tears evaporate more quickly. Our tears keep our eyes sharp, clean, hydrated and glossy. Dry eyes can cause redness, itching and an accumulation of grit, which may contribute to blurriness and eyesight. Shugarman tells us, "The pupils get smaller, muscles in the eye adjust the size of the lens, and the two eyes have to converge. To remedy this problem, look away from the screen a few times an hour to give eye muscles a break and avoid strain.

Do you have Brain Freeze, Brain Fog, or Brain Farts? A recent study in China showed that too much internet use could cause structural damage to your brain. "The researchers studied 17 adolescents with Internet Addiction Disorder (IAD) and found structural and functional interference in the part of the brain that regulates organization, possibly causing cognitive impairment similar to that caused by gambling and alcoholism." The study findings show that "those that abused the bright lights of technology had abnormal white matter integrity in brain regions involved in emotional generation and processing, executive attention, decision making and cognitive control", write the authors.

"Your Energized Bunny" keeps going, going, and going
EMF Kids on Krack

The "less you burn, better health you will earn." When you turn off the juice, there is less abuse. Children's brains are much more sensitive to the Electro Magnetic Field (EMF) than we think. We need to remember that their brains are still developing and can be damaged by being bombarded with frequent EMF impulses. EMF is not just with cell phones, iPods, and iPads, but with microwaves, indoor lighting, and on a larger scale, outdoor street lights, satellite dishes, satellite towers, GPS...everything...It's electric. Did you ever thin about the headphones kids have plugged into their phones, little antennas transmitting frequencies directly to their brain? Some kids sleep with their phones right next to their heads or have a clock radio in close proximity allowing a nightly supply of EMF's to have a "sleepover in their brain."

There is the case of 21-year-old Tiffany Frantz from Pennsylvania who slipped her cell phone into her bra 12 hours a day for 5 years. She noticed a small lump in her breast and was diagnosed with breast cancer. She had a mastectomy on her left breast, which is where she kept her phone. Coincidence?

In today's world, it is crazy not to intervene and restrict or limit the technology. The nervous system is hyped up...making it harder for your child to get to sleep from the stream of frequencies buzzing through their body. The health effects from abuse of EMF include decreased immune function, increased blood pressure, impaired nervous system function, cancers and brain damage.

How About Good Energy?

Did you know that everything has energy? Quantum physics shows us that everything has a different amount of energy, and this energy can be either good or bad. Quantum physics is the study of the behavior of matter and energy at the molecular, atomic, nuclear, and even smaller microscopic levels. The birth of quantum physics is attributed to Max Planck's 1900 paper on blackbody radiation. Development of the field was done by Max Planck, Albert Einstein and many other scientists. Energy is real!

There is an energy test called QRA, Quantum Reflex Analysis. I am sure some of you have heard of kinesiology, which is a similar energy test. Being a QRA practitioner, I can test everything and anything from the body's organs, food, glass, stone, dirt, even clothes to see if the energy is good or bad. If I test glass, it has a very strong energy, but when I test a plastic bag it has a very bad energy.

Your Body Can Talk to You?

What if your body could talk to you and tell you what was wrong and what you needed to be healthy? Did you know that it could through Quantum Reflex Analysis (QRA), a unique, highly effective testing of the bio-energetic status of the body's key organs and glands? It uses a university proven muscle-testing technique of medically accepted reflex points. QRA can quickly pinpoint problem areas to determine the precise nutrients and exact amounts needed to rapidly restore your energy and dramatically improve your health. It has the ability to identify and eliminate the "root of the problem." Practitioners use specific testing techniques to identify hidden infections that may be causing ill health from interference sites from traumas, surgeries, improper eating habits, stress, etc. In just one session, your practitioner can determine what key organs are deficient and provide you with an overall assessment and program to get you started on a new state of health.

You will learn how your individual body communicates its needs through the language of QRA. Our bodies have a magnificent internal intelligence that can rejuvenate the body and return the endurance, vitality, peak mental and physical performance and health that we all enjoyed in our younger years. Your body can talk to you through an amazing bio-communication technique called QRA. It includes specific testing techniques to find hidden infections, hormone imbalance, thyroid imbalance, digestive problems, skin rashes, and heart trouble, just to name a few. QRA can also find deficiencies in vitamins such as B, D and Calcium. Your QRA Practitioner will test acupuncture meridians on the surface of your body. You will need to have strength in your hands or call your practitioner ahead of time so that they may provide a surrogate to help assist during the test. You will be asked to create an "O-ring" with your fingers and place a finger of your other hand directly onto the acupuncture meridian point(s). This technique is painless, simple and easy to perform. Once the practitioner has determined which organs/glands need help, they will test nutrients or formulas to find the exact match your body needs. Your body will actually pick the supplements and the amounts needed to nourish unhealthy organs and glands back to health. I have treated over 200 chronically ill, fatigued, and diseased patients, teaching everyone the secrets of regeneration and healing though organic supplementation, external detoxing and proper nutrition. **To find a QRA practitioner in your area, call Premier Research Labs at 800-370-3447.**

How Can I Protect My Kids and Myself? "You Can't See the Winds, but You Can Feel the Effects of the Wind"

There is a company called Premier Research Labs that carry devices for your protection from the effects of EMF. Premier offers a Q-Disc, which is an ultra-thin polarity disc for all mobile phones, including iPhones. You simply install this device on the back of your phone for your daily protection. I have a Q-Disc on my phone and keep it near me when I work on my computer for extra protection. Did you know that a 30-second cell phone call can weaken every cell in your body? The Q-Disk protects you from the EMFs and converts the harmful field into a beneficial field.

Also, I recommend the Pyra Fire Pyramid, also from Premier for home, business and car use. This pyramid creates a strong coherent field, which transforms the depolarizing energy into a healing, beneficial energy that strengthens and protects us from all EMFs. I bring one in the car, and on airplanes, and especially when I stay in a hotel, where the room is buzzing with all types of interference. You are not only protecting yourself from the EFA effects, you are changing the energy into a more peaceful environment. When people come into my center, they remark about how good it feels. This is amazing that even people that do not understand energy can feel the effects of it. This is an important purchase that you need to make to continue your health journey.

10

"*ANGRY BIRDS*" NEGATIVE EFFECTS FROM TV, MOVIES, GAMES

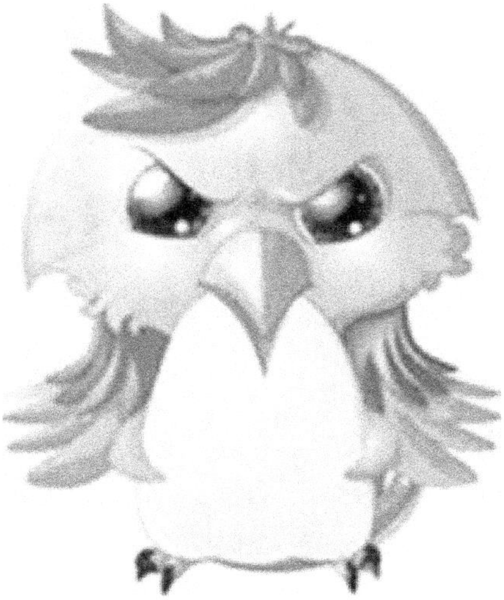

Let's face it, kids today are glued to the tube, movies and the internet. Who doesn't ask *Alexa* or Ok *Google* for jokes, trivia, sports scores, directions and even recipes? It is just the way of life in today's world. It also becomes the teacher for our kids and even molds their behaviors and moods. If you try to ask a question when your child is watching TV, you may not get an answer because they are so absorbed. They seem likes "boobs at the tube", zombie kids, mesmerized by the dazzling display of lights, actions, vivid music, etc. They do not have to use their imagination or think because all of the answers are there for them. They seem to withdraw into their own little world for hours; they do not need anyone or anything. Many psychologists are concerned that children are daydreaming more but losing their creative ideas and imagination.

Don't get me wrong, Dora and Barney are helpful at school age but how about the violence that has become mainstream? Blood, violence and the thrill of "to kill or be killed" is destroying our world.

Violence – a Learned Behavior

Many believe that violence and aggression is a learned behavior and can be learned from media. Adults and kids learn new ways to be aggressive and incorporate it into their daily lives. People get desensitized, so the more they watch, it seems to be conceived as "not as bad", "not as bloody", "not as scary." When they get angry, irritated, or frustrated, they may impulsively put these negative behaviors to actual use in assaults against others. Kids seem to think that violence is an acceptable way to handle problems and issues with others. Your kids feel they are invincible like superheroes, especially watching their superheroes who never die.

How Much TV Do Kids Watch?

Children aged 2 to 11 watch approximately 28 hours of television per week. Other surveys suggest that the number is about 35 hours a week. This does not include internet games and movies.

Where do They Watch Violence?

- Prime Time Series - little or no violence
- Network movies - some violence
- Theatrical Films had significantly more violence
- Saturday Morning Cartoons received mixed reviews of violence. Mighty Morphins Power Rangers, X-Men were most popular but contained violence
- Premium cable channels – show the most violence
- Violent Video Games – score high in violence
- Movie Theatres – R rated movies, the most succesful movies contain high amounts of violence

"Researchers termed the action in these programs as "Sinister Combat Violence" because they are obsessed primarily with violence, the whole story line leads to violence, and the main characters are always pre-occupied with using violence to get their ways."

Negative Effects of Television Violence

- Imitate the violence they observe on TV
- Children become "immune" to the horror of violence
- May accept violence as a way to solve problems
- Identify with certain TV characters and superheroes
- Media provides a false view of reality

School Shootings

Let's not forget that horrific day on April 20, 1999 when two school students, Eric Harris and Dylan Klebold, dressed in trench coats, began shooting fellow students outside Columbine High School. Today, school shootings have escalated with real life violence, where many kids were fans of violent games and movies.

Here's a list of the mass murders linked with video games:

1. Adam Lanza walked into Sandy Hook Elementary, Connecticut in 2012; he was a frequent player of violent first-person shooter video games for long hours every day in his bedroom.
2. James Holmes went on a shooting rampage in a movie theater showing *The Dark Knight Rises* in Colorado in 2012. Holmes frequently played of violent video games including World of Warcraft, an infamously addictive role-playing game.
3. Jared Lee Loughner of Tucson, shot Rep. Gabrielle Giffords and killed six others in 2011. He was both mentally ill and a video gamer.
4. Eric Harris had no contempt for others and his total lack of empathy and conscience is evidence of his psychopathic tendencies during a high school shooting in Colorado,, 1999. He also enjoyed violent video games.
5. Elliot Rodger, killed seven young men and women, including himself in 2011 in California. He was hooked on violent video games from a young age. He felt comfortable and secure hiding himself in *World of Warcraft*.

6. Nehemiah Griego, killed five, including his mother, father and his three younger siblings. New Mexico 2013. He loved playing violent video games and even enjoyed talking about them to crime investigators.
7. Jacob Tyler Roberts, played violent video games. His rampage renacted a violent scene from *Grand Theft Auto* in 2012 in Oregon.
8. Anders Behring Breivik shot 68 people dead in 2011 at a youth camp of the Norwegian Labor party, another nine in a bombing of government buildings. He liked playing violent games and used the video game *Call of Duty* to train for his shooting massacre.
9. Michael Carneal shot girls as they prayed in a prayer group in 1997 in Kentucky. Carneal never moved his feet during his shootings, and never fired far to the left or right, but instead fired only once at each target that appeared, just as a player of video games maximizes his game score by shooting only once at each victim, in order to hit as many targets as possible.
10. Jose Reyes, a 12-year-old boy, opened fire with a semiautomatic handgun at Sparks Middle School, in Nevada. He killed a teacher and wounded two students before turning the gun on himself in 2013. He had watched violent video games for months.
11. Dylann Storm Roof, killed nine black churchgoers in South Carolina during a Bible study in 2015. He spent much of his time playing violent video games.
12. Jeff Weise, a 16-year-old, killed nine people near his high school in Red Lake, Minnesota in 2015. Weise had an obsession with violent animation.
13. Chris Harper-Mercer, killed nine people and another seven were injured from his shooting that took place at a community college in southern Oregon.
14. Evan Ramsey, snuck a shot gun into his Alaska high school in 1997 and shot a student and the principal and wounded two others. He claims that a video game, Doom, distorted his version of reality, "I did not understand that if I pull out a gun and shoot you ... you're not getting back up".

Parents need to pay close attention to their kids to make sure to watch age appropriate shows. As children grow, their curious nature and pressure from what other friends are watching will be very challenging for you and your child. We need to understand that tv puts images of violence into their impressionable brains. If your kids are fed violence from video games and violent movies, they will have the need and stimulation to watch more. The "older they get, the harder they fall", and the harder it will be to control their "out of control" addiciton to stimuli from violence. If you look at the top selling movies today, the main theme for most is violence.

Solutions to Help Reduce Violence

- Pay attention to the programs your kids are watching
- Watch TV and movies with them
- Be selective of games you are purchasing
- Set limits on the amount of time spent with television
- Incorporate other activities instead of media
- Be realistic and explain that actors, superheroes, and game characters will live but in real life people will die
- Explain how wrong violence is and the consequences
- Disapprove of violence and explain how to problem solve by talking and safe ways to express anger.
- Contact parents of their friends and enforce similar rules and movie and game choices.

11

"GOOSEBUMPS" RELAXATION FOR KIDS

It is a great idea to teach relaxation techniques starting with very young children to reduce stress.

1. **"Blow them away" Deep Breathing techniques**

   Deep breathing is an effective way of slowing down the body's natural response to stress. It slows down the heart rate, lowers blood pressure and provides a feeling of being in control.

   Tell your kids we are going to play a game and they will not even know they are doing relaxation techniques. Make sure you do this with them. Tell them we are playing the Supergirl or Superman game.

Supergirl or Superman - super hero powers of wind game

Sit Down, feet on the floor, sitting up straight
Simply breathe in deeply to the count of 10
Hold the breath for a moment to the count of 5
Release it slowly to the count of 10
Repeat the deep breathing until you feel relaxed.

2. **Progressive Muscle Relaxation**

   Progressive muscle relaxation offers a wonderful way to relieve stress. This is accomplished by tensing and then relaxing different muscle groups in your body.

The Green Lantern Game

Buy a green ring. Put the ring on your child and tell them they are going to recharge their body like the Green Lantern has to. Sit across from your child and have them do what you do. We will be tensing the entire body starting with your face and adding many other body muscles. At the end you will be holding all of the muscles at once.

a. Scrunch up your face with a face freeze and hold
b. Bring your shoulders up to your ears and hold
c. Make a fist with your hands and hold
d. Tense up your shoulders
e. Pull in your belly and hold
f. Stretch out your legs and tighten up the leg muscles and hold
g. Point your toes and hold

Next relax, hold up your hand that wears the ring and repeat the Oath three times "In brightest day, in blackest night, No evil shall escape my sight. Let those who worship evil's might, Beware my power--Green Lantern's light!"

3. **Exercise**

   Swimming - Aquaman has super strength, exceptional swimming skills, and the ability to breathe underwater. Buy an Aquaman patch, t-shirt or button for your child to wear. Limit swimming, your child's skin is absorbing the chorine. Try to use pools that are treated with salt.
   Speed Running – Tell your little kids you are going to be running at the speed of sound like the superhero Flash. Buy a Flash t-shirt, a lightning bolt, a watch or even better a Fitbit so he can chart his steps.

See an extensive list of exercise selections in Chapter 4, ADHD.

4. **Visualization**

   This is also known as guided imagery. This technique is wonderful for kids since it uses the imagination to slow down the chatter of the mind and help release negative thoughts and worries. The following is fun and relaxing for both you and your child.

Visualization – you will need to buy 7 colors of stones, or if you can't find stones crayons will do. You could also do an art project and make things in the following colors: red, orange, yellow, blue, green, purple, and lavender.

Also, buy some lavender essential oils from a health food store for the beginning and end of the visualization.

a. Have your child sit across from you
b. Place a drop of lavender in the palms of their hands and yours, rub together
c. Close your eyes and take three deep breaths of the lavender
d. Tell them to open their eyes
e. Start to read the visualization and when you get to the color, hand your child that color to hold and look at.
f. Read in a soft calm voice

Give them the color red and have them stare at it. Feel the warmth and energy from the color red. Look at the red crayon or object. Feel the sun is directly overhead and you feel the brightness and warmth from the top of your head and throughout your body. Red gives you courage and makes you feel strong. Now breathe in the color red and as you inhale, feel the intense power of red. As you exhale, breathe out any fears and doubts you may have about yourself.

Now pick up orange - Become the color orange. Orange is a joyful color. You feel very happy inside. Imagine eating a healthy sweet juicy orange. Perhaps you see a beautiful orange butterfly. You feel light, giggly! Inhale orange and breathe in happiness and joy. As you exhale breathe out bad habits and sadness.

Now pick up yellow - Breathe in the color yellow and breathe in confidence in yourself. Become a yellow happy face or a happy minion. Imagine a pretty yellow bird on a yellow sunflower. Breathe in the color yellow, breathe in self-worth and fun, and exhale your worries and stress.

Now pick up green - Breathe in the color green and breathe in the color of harmony and balance and peace. Feel the strength from the green lantern. Smell the fresh green grass and trees, eat a fresh juicy green apple. Breathe in green and breathe in peace and good health, exhale sickness and hatred.

Now pick up blue - Breathe in the color blue and breathe in your creativity and communication. Become a blue Smurf and know how easy it is to talk to others in the village. Look at the beautiful blue sky, with the white fluffy clouds. Inhale the color blue and breathe in truthfulness and creativity and exhale dishonesty and shyness.

Now pick up purple - Breathe in the color purple and breathe in your inner voice. Learn to listen to the voice that says "go for it." Become purple like Barney or a purple Care Bear or my Pretty Pony. Taste the sweetness of purple grapes or the smell of purple lavender flowers. Breathe in purple and trust what you are feeling and exhale depression.

Now pick up lavender - Breathe in the color lavender and breathe in faith. No matter how bad things get we always have hope and faith. Imagine wellness, goodness, happiness and love. Imagine letting go of some lavender balloons and watching them float into the sky. Breathe in lightness and gratitude and breathe out negativity.

Now give your child all the colored stones of red, orange, yellow, green, blue, purple, lavender. They have now collected seven powerful healing colors, their personal rainbow. Whenever they wish to feel calm, refreshed and balanced, meditate on these colorful vibrations.

End with a lavender inhalation with three deep breaths.

5. **Laughter**

Laughter is a wonderful stress reliever and can bring happiness and joy into your child's life. It can change a child's mood within minutes.

Ways to encourage your child to laugh include:

- Make funny faces
- Play peek a boo
- Say funny words like butt
- Watch a funny movie or cartoon
- Watch old slapstick shows like the three stooges. Kids love when people fall down.
- Make up a joke
- Jump on the bed
- Have a pillow fight
- A good ole tickle
- Read a funny book
- Make a fart sound
- Make a burping sound
- Dress up in silly costumes
- Blow bubbles
- Dance around

The freeze game - stay in a pose and don't move. Let them pick and poke at you and then jump out and yell!

No talking game - especially in the car. The winner is the last one to stay quiet. They will be laughing in no time.

6. **Stretch & Yoga**

Kids and teens can enjoy yoga poses, which offer lots of gentile stretching, and breathing exercises that can be incorporated into their everyday life. Yoga is used to achieve peacefulness of body and mind, helping you relax and manage stress and anxiety. Young kids will enjoy the animal yoga poses. For small kids, give them a toy animal for the pose they are doing.

- Cobra
- Frog
- Half Lotus
- Downward facing dog
- Up dog
- Plank or turtle
- Forward bend or giraffe pose
- Warrior or wide winged pose
- Chair or sitting bear pose
- Tree or flamingo pose
- Plow or panda bear pose
- Cat
- Cow
- Happy Baby
- Fish
- Eagle

Go to: ***27 Yoga Positions Demonstrated by Animals***

https://www.buzzfeed.com/whitneyjefferson/the-animal-guide-to-yoga?utm_term=.xmYjAxKrp0#.vd20GwY4Zq

7. **Listen to Music**

   You can "crank up the volume" and "twist and shout", twirl and spin and get rid of the stress. Using nature sounds and new age music can be very relaxing to help calm down and de-stress your child. Enya, Kitaro, Yanni and George Winston are a few of my favorites.

   When doing homework, some kids do better with a distraction, especially those with ADHD/ADD. Ask them which type of music they would like.

8. **Meditate**

   Stay in the moment and learn how to slow down the intense whirlwind of stress by embracing meditation. These skills can weave together your own path to a strong mind/body/spirit connection. Meditation helps us to stay focused and stay in the moment, meaning not dwelling on the past or worrying about the future.

"Yesterday is history, tomorrow is a mystery, and today is a gift of God, which is why we call it a present", Bill Keane

When I was 15 years old, I had the wonderful opportunity of learning from a Maharishi how to do transcendental meditation. I had such a traumatic life filled with stress, that I immediately embraced meditation. I met privately with the Maharishi who gave me a mantra, a sound that has no association to a word, to use with my meditation. The first time I meditated, I had this sensation in my brain, a release I have never felt before in my life. I was hooked immediately, on "a good thing" early in my life.

Meditation is a safe and simple way to balance a person's physical, emotional, and mental states. It is easily learned and has been used as an aid in treating stress, pain management, hypertension and heart disease. Meditation has been practiced for several thousand years. Today, the science of meditation proves through extensive studies that the frontal lobe of the brain goes offline, the thalamus reduces the flow of incoming information to a trickle, and the parietal lobe slows down. Studies have shown that a person that meditates actually has lower blood pressure, uses 17% less oxygen, lowered heart rates by three beats a minute and increases their theta brain waves (the ones that appear right before sleep).

The purpose of meditation is to calm our mind so we can enjoy some peacefulness. People who meditate find that they worry less and are much happier. Meditation does not have to be complex. It tones and tunes up the thinking processes and the emotions and brings everyday life into sharper focus with new degrees of ease and harmony. Meditation requires nothing on your part but the time it takes to do it.

There are so many types of meditation. There are Breath Meditations, Transcendental Meditation (TM) mantra meditations, walking meditations, and guided meditations. All meditations have a few things in common; we need to focus on something such as a word, mantra (sound), ocean waves or breath. Then when our mind starts to wander we slowly come back to our breath or sound. When using a mantra, we come back by thinking of that sound repeatedly. During meditation, we try to ignore all of the distractions around us: noise in our head, talking, cars outside, or even the clock. As we become more advanced, we will meditate and not even hear the many of the distractions, especially those in our mind.

It is best not to eat before meditation, but if you are hungry try a nutrition bar or piece of fruit. When meditating at home, try to create a peaceful atmosphere by disconnecting your phone, closing your door for privacy, and putting any animals out of the room.

Adult and Teen Meditation

1. Find a quiet place, turn out the lights, sit comfortably in a chair, lying is not recommended since many people tend to fall asleep instead of meditating.
2. Rub some lavender between your palms and inhale with three deep breaths.
3. Close your eyes and shut out the world; begin to relax the muscles in your body.
4. Next breathe naturally, preferably through the nostrils inhaling and exhaling.
5. Just continue to follow your breath, becoming aware of the sensation of the breath as it enters and leaves the nostrils. If you prefer to use a sound, you can use the universal sound of "om" as your mantra.
6. In the beginning, you will be more aware you are meditating, our minds may be very busy, we feel distracted. Thoughts and distractions, including worries, our kids, things we need to be doing, disagreements with friends, and noises outside will enter our mind. Once we realize that we are distracting, we can gently bring ourselves back to the meditation and start to follow our breath or repeat the "om" sound silently. The more we practice, the more patient and relaxed we will become. Our mind will feel clear, spacious, and refreshed. Eventually meditation will become more natural and we will be thinking less and not notice our distractions.
7. I usually practice meditation for twenty minutes daily. It is best to start out small and work up to longer sessions. It is recommended to meditate twice a day, once in the morning and again in the early evening.

Children's Meditation

1. For children simply put Ocean waves on
2. Sit on the bed with your legs straight out, with a couple pillows behind you

3. Stretch your arms over your head and stretch
4. Try to touch your toes sitting
5. Rub your hands with lavender and breathe in three times
6. Tell your child to close their eyes
7. Tell your child to breathe in and out
8. Tell them to envision they are at the beach
9. Tell them we are going to play the quiet game for two minutes
10. Start with two minutes and start to increase the time by 1-minute every time until reaching 20 minutes
11. End with another stretch over your head
12. Pick another essential oil such as peppermint or lemon to wake up

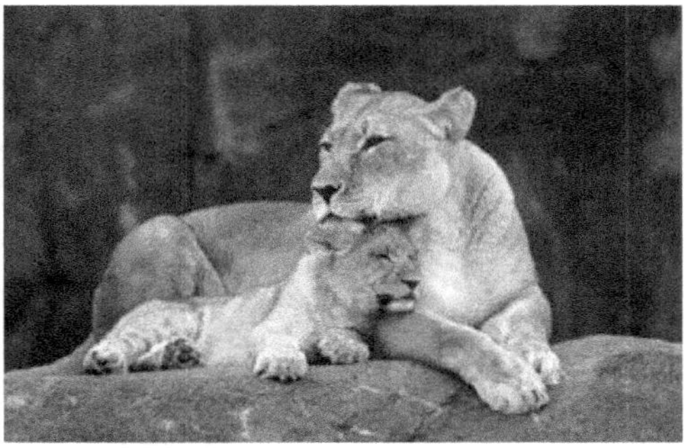

9. Snuggle Science

We all need to get our Hugging, Snuggling, Cuddling time in. Even Donkey in Shrek says "I can't feel my toes; I think I need a hug." We know it feels good, but did you know there is science backing that feeling? We all love holding hands and being touched because it releases a cocktail of neurotransmitters in our brain including serotonin, dopamine and oxytocin. Research has shown that a loving touch boosts our immune system; reduces stress, anxiety and fears, fights depression, boosts our moods; lowers our blood pressure; lowers heart rates and even regenerates muscle tissue in mice. So what happens when you get scared during a horror flick? Do you reach out and touch someone? Take time to snuggle together! Let your child snuggle with stuffed animals and definitely with real animals as well.

10. **Hypnotherapy for Teens and Children that can Follow Directions**

Teens have a concoction of brewing stressors such as: decision-making, more responsibility and an increase of raging hormones racing through their bodies. Male or female, they worry about school tests, fitting in with friends, acne breakouts and their weight. Most teens spend a lot of their time in school where they are not taught how to deal with their life stressors. Teens are pushed to the limits and they need time to relax.

There are many issues where hypnotherapy can help since many of them stem from unresolved emotional issues and stress. Hypnosis can help with:

- Asthma
- Allergies
- Aggression
- Nail biting
- Stuttering
- Fears
- Study habits
- Public speaking
- Anger
- Concentration
- Lose weight

Hypnosis is a trance like state of mind, which is used to help a person gain more control over behaviors, emotions and physical well-being. It is also helpful with addictions such as quitting smoking, drugs, and overeating. The difference between counseling is that instead of trying to get children to talk, we find the root problems and let them relax while giving them positive suggestions to make improvements.

11. Massage (kids, teens, pregnancy)

Massage is great as a reward for a job well done, or to relieve stress from a hard day at school. Children hold their stress in their shoulders, which can cause a lot of pain in their backs making it difficult to relax. Young athletes can benefit with a sports massage, helping to alleviate discomfort and recover much faster from injuries. Most of all, visiting the spa or massage therapist is just a place that kids and teens can go for instant relief from stress.

Pregnancy Massage

Massage can help you prepare for the birthing process in several ways:

a. Release chronic tension in lower back, abdomen & inner thighs
b. Increase your awareness of tension & teaches you to consciously release
c. Increase your sense of confidence & self-control
d. Practice focus & relaxation breathing techniques during your massage

Just taking time out for a massage can improve your outlook in life, making everything seem easier during this time of many changes.

Benefits of Massage

- Produces natural chemicals in the brain
- Pain-relieving properties
- Euphoria, appetite modulation, healthy immune
- Relaxes muscles, can correct damaged muscles
- Improves circulation without increasing heart load
- Increases range of motion
- Helps obtain a feeling of connectedness
- Relieves pain from muscle tension, fractures, sprains, sciatica, and stiff joints
- Shortens recovery time from muscular strain
- Flushes lactic acid, uric acid and other metabolic wastes from tissues
- Stretches the ligaments and tendons, keeping them supple
- Stimulates the skin and nervous system while relaxing the nerves
- Helps reduce emotional and physical stress

12

"HOW TO TRAIN YOUR DRAGON" - DISCIPLINE

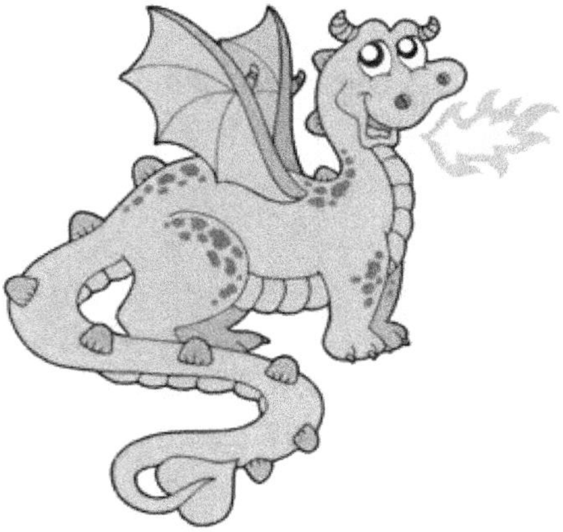

We can pray, search for Harry Potters magic wand, wish upon Geppetto's star, find Aladdin's genie, wear Dorothy's ruby slippers, or plant some magic beans, anything to help find the perfect discipline for our children. The word discipline means to teach and instill knowledge and skill. This is our way to protect our children from harm.

Parents are often confused about how to discipline their children. Many parents think of discipline as punishment, power and control where others are afraid to introduce any type of discipline. Parents are searching for the perfect balance, the best and most effective ways. Parents are not only confused about too much or too little but also how to set limits with their kids. The ultimate goal is to help their child develop great self-esteem and self-control.

Parents have different ideas about discipline depending on how they were raised. Some parents were raised very lenient, some very strict and some a combination between the two. Then it gets even more complicated when you have to define strict or lenient and work through your differences. You and your partner might find it difficult agreeing on how to raise you kids. You learned from different parents with different techniques. Many parents will pick a technique that is the opposite of how they were raised, which changes with every generation. I was raised in an alcoholic family, so when I raised my son I was especially affectionate and supportive since I felt ignored and abandoned. It is important for you to talk extensively about how you would like to raise your children, looking at the pros and cons to create the very best plan for your family. Compromise is essential between parents to find the harmony needed for a stable relationship between you and your children. Some couples may need to find a counselor to help them work out their difference. Remember when we react to a situation with anger, we are really reacting to something that happened in our past. It strikes a nerve and we become angry because it is a reminder of an uncomfortable situation, not really the situation at hand. Some couples may need individual counseling to work out issues from their own childhood.

Three Main Types of Parenting: Authoritative, Authoritarian and Permissive.

An **authoritative parent** is the most effective type of parenting. It has clear expectations and consequences and is affectionate and loving towards children. If the right type of discipline is started very early, your child will glide into the relationship feeling loved and safe. They will know very early on who the parent is and who the child is. The authoritative parent allows for flexibility and collaborative problem solving with the child when dealing with behavioral challenges. The purpose of effective discipline is to help children organize themselves, internalize rules and acquire appropriate behavior patterns and age appropriate expectations. Good discipline gives children a greater trust between the child and the parent.

Good parenting is learning to set limits at an early age. The longer you wait the harder it is. Kids feel safer when they know their parents have a different role and that they are in charge. Parents and kids need to feel respected to have a healthy relationship. Kids want limits, schedules, and routine. This makes them feel safe.

Healthy discipline with mutual respect is a firm, fair and consistent way. The goal is to protect your child from danger, help your child learn self-discipline, and develop a healthy sense of responsibility and control.

Authoritarian parenting is a less effective type of parenting. It does have clear expectations and consequences, but shows little affection toward the child. Strict parenting can come from growing up in a strict family. Strictness can come from very hostile families, growing up in an addictive or abusive family and are often prone to extreme disciplinary measures toward their children. These families rarely express their feelings or tell one another that they love them. Parents who were raised in these environments pass on to their kids, their cold, angry personalities. These learned habits can surface with their own children; they may ignore, reject or disapprove of them as a result.

Strict parenting may control behavior temporarily but it does not help the child to self-discipline and become responsible for themselves. Children become focused on the negative aspects of being yelled at or spanked, and become numb, resistant, resentful and angry. The **more power and control you use, the more out of control they become**. This type of parenting is based on fear, power and control and teaches a child to become a bully and grow up to use force in their own lives especially with children. Our children will mimic our behaviors; with force you get force and with yelling you get yelling. When this war develops, the fighting will escalate as your child ages.

Many of the children raised in fear, negativity, violence and yelling become depressed. Because they are always being yelled at they are taught they are "no good" that something is wrong with them. Depression mixed with low self-esteem turns these kids into loners. Harsh discipline such as humiliation (verbal abuse, shouting, and name-calling) will also make it hard for the child to respect and trust the parent. They may be compliant but feel unable to cope with life in a healthy way. They are not able to think for themselves; they learn that the only way to communicate is with power, by being rebellious, angry and through aggression. Others are the opposite, take on a more passive aggressive behavior, and become followers. They do not take responsibility for their actions. Later in life, they overreact to criticism reverting back to the way they were criticized or told what to do when they were younger. They also try to build themselves up anyway they can by fabricating stories. They have a hard time with relationships with friends and partners since they were never taught emotional development, love and empathy. Strict discipline does not help your kids behave; it is based on negativity and takes all of the positivity out of the equation.

"Who's the Boss" Permissive Parenting

A **permissive parent** is the least effective form of parenting. They show a lot of affection toward their child but provide little discipline. Children will miss one of the most important lessons they need to learn; learning how to manage themselves and to handle or tolerate frustration. When a child does not learn how to be frustrated, sad or angry, they do not learn internal happiness because these feelings are being avoided and the child may feel unacceptable. Many children that get their way and are raised permissively are referred to as being spoiled and very self-centered. Children learn that their disappointments and sadness are intolerable and that their parents will do almost anything to avoid letting them feel disappointed. Children, who grow up sheltered, grow up in fear of what disappointment and frustration is, thinking they are unbearable. Children raised without reasonable limits will have difficulty adjusting socially. Permissive children that are used to getting their way may cheat to win to avoid what they have been taught, to not be disappointed.

Permissive parents make constant compromises letting their child get away with things and even treat them badly. This creates a hostile relationship between the two, which gets worse over time. A parent will become angry and resentful from the child and can start to pull away from nurturing the child with love and attention. Kids begin to distrust their parents because of the constant caving, being wishy washy and not showing strength. The child will continue to look for more challenging events and start pushing the limits.

If parents were raised in a very independent family themselves, they may be uncomfortable in enforcing rules and setting limits. They hope that their children will learn from their mistakes instead of teaching them. If parents were raised without love and attention, they may choose to give unconditional love, which to them means constantly showing affection to their children. One or both parents may offer "too much love" and start to smother their children and they grow up immature and wanting others to take care of them. Finding this perfect medium can be quite a challenge. Families that lean towards being overly affectionate seem to be more accepting of the child and don't openly show their children their mistakes. These kids feel they can do no wrong. Some parents feel that have to do everything for the child, because maybe they feel their parents did not do enough for them. This teaches the child they cannot do things on their own and again, encourage laziness, shyness and dependencies.

Children who become the boss at such an early age will not understand when they are older why their parents are starting to TRY to discipline them. At this point, they have been so used to getting their way that a constant struggle for power will develop. Children that are not disciplined grow up controlling the parents and are accustomed to always getting what they want. It is imperative to set limits. If limits are not established, the relationships they will form later in life with teachers, friends, lovers and even employers will be in jeopardy. They will still try to have it their way by throwing adult tantrums; more times than none, these tantrums will end in failed relationships. We used to sing the Rolling Stones song *You Can't Always get What you Want* with our kids, which would actually get a smile.

Discipline for Newborns – Eating, Sleeping, Peeing and Pooping

Infants need a schedule around feeding, sleeping, play and interaction with others. The schedule helps regulate a sense of predictability, a way to help them feel safe. They cry to let us know their needs, if they are hungry, tired or need a diaper change. However, babies learn very early how to turn their needs into wants. Remember discipline is about teaching your child and it is recommended to start as early as a few months old. Here is where many parents think they need to wait until their children are older. They think they are too young or need to understand verbally what you are saying before any type of discipline is started. Children understand how to communicate when they are babies. Their wants and needs are the same thing. If they want something and cry to show us they are hungry or need changing, they are already letting us know they need us. They understand that when they cry they will get a response. If this continues when they are older, they will use the same technique that has worked their entire life and will cry to see what they can get.

Infants should not be overstimulated. They should be allowed to develop some tolerance to frustration and the ability to self-soothe. Discipline should not involve techniques such as time-out (see Forms of discipline), spanking or consequences. "Setting limits is a critical part of your responsibility as a parent," says Claire Lerner, LCSW, director of parenting resources at Zero to Three, in Washington, D.C. You're helping your child to understand right and wrong, to follow rules, and to cope with frustration and disappointment. Of course, we all know that a baby who is "misbehaving" isn't doing so intentionally. When she tugs at your glasses, she's simply doing her job -- exploring the world around her. "Babies are constantly making observations about the world," says Harvey Karp, MD, author of *The Happiest Toddler on the Block* (Bantam). "She mushes her food to see how it feels. She drops something from the high chair to see how it splats."

Discipline at 4 to 7 Months

At this stage, you can start differentiating between needs and wants. Your baby may **want** to fall asleep in your lap, but they do not **need** to...they need to fall asleep on their own. It is recommended to sleep in their own crib in their own room, to not develop a dependent relationship.

Babies are curious at this age and learn by exploring. They start to grab at things looking for reactions. It is actually worse to react by saying no or ouch because at this age it may be more fun for them. When they get a reaction, they will start to do this repeatedly to get a response. It is best to put the child down and say nothing. Teething and biting can also be a problem at this age, especially with breastfeeding. It has been recommended to gently push baby closer to your breast instead of reacting.

Discipline at 7 to 12 Months

This is the crucial time to childproof your home. You can set up; gates, install light socket covers, and especially the "child proof" latches on kitchen cabinets. Remove all toxic cleaners and store up high to protect your kids. It is important for toddlers to start to experiment with control and exercising their own will. If your child is around something dangerous, you will need to remove the child or the object, give them a firm "No – hot", and redirect them to an alternative activity or toy. It is a great idea to have one cabinet open in the kitchen filled with their toys so they have something that is not off limits.

At the early toddler stage, it is normal and necessary for toddlers to experiment with control of the physical world and with the capacity to exercise their own will versus that of others. Consequently, parental tolerance is recommended. Disciplinary interventions are necessary to ensure the toddler's safety, limit aggression, and prevent destructive behavior.

In addition, this is a time when children suffer from separation anxiety. At this age, we want to let them play on their own. If we leave the room, take a little time to come back. Use a reassuring voice saying you are there. Running right back, picking them up constantly when they cry, just lets them know they will get whatever they want whenever they want. Kids are too young and should not be kept in time-out away from the parent.

Discipline at 12 to 18 Months

Children like to test their vocal cords at this age. It is best not to laugh or yell when they do this. Try using a firm but soothing voice and tell them we do not use a loud voice here. It is important to take your children to church, restaurant, etc. They need to learn how to behave in different environments. When you visit a restaurant, bring toys for them to play with. Unfortunately, you will need to continuously explain the rules. They do not have a lot of self-control, but how you handle them now will help to set them up for good behavior in a few months. If you let them get away with yelling at inappropriate places, they will continue to do this whenever they feel the need for attention. Some parents do not bring their children out at all, and they do not learn how to behave out in public. When children misbehave at this age, it is very important to correct behavior. If you give a child what they want when they cry, they will play you every time. They learn this is how I behave to get what I want. If you do not give in, they will learn that if they misbehave they will get nothing. It is our responsibility to teach them the difference between right and wrong. If we give in...they do not learn. If they want to go outside instead of eating dinner, they know all they have to do is cry and it will happen. The longer we submit to this behavior, the harder it will be to correct it. Many parents hate to upset their kids, hear them cry, see them angry or endure a tantrum. We also come home tired and it seems so easy to just give in and let them have their way. It is important for parents to develop good parenting by setting limits, being consistent and following a routine, especially when eating and at bedtime, the same time every night.

Discipline at 18 to 24 Months: Autonomy and Rebellion

Children start to learn language and become cute little chatterboxes. They have a hard time expressing their feelings at this age. We are needed to help them to understand by explaining to them when they feel frustrated. They have a strong need to do things on their own; they don't want you to do things for them. If they cannot do something, you can help them, and explain what you are doing to help them. If they are having trouble with a puzzle, you can explain to them "let me help you, see you turn it this way."

Children also start to hit and bite. Here we must be firm and let them know this is an undesirable behavior. You need to remove them from the situation and tell them firmly, "No", then explain to them why, "because it hurts". Children become very frustrated at this age so pay special attention to what is upsetting them. Singing and pretend voices are a great way to help children behave. It your child wants to do something that is dangerous, like try to open a gate, redirect and start singing a little song or use a pretend voice (high pitch or very low voice.)

Early toddlers are not verbal enough to understand or mature enough to respond to verbal prohibitions. Verbal directions and explanations are unreliable forms of discipline for early toddlers

Parents must learn to be consistent even when everyday pressure comes into our lives: we feel tired, overwhelmed with finances, illness, etc. It makes it easy to go back and forth between showing warmth and becoming hostile. This sends mixed messages to your child. It is imperative not to show your differences, drama or arguments around your children. With parenting, it is important to stay consistent with your discipline allowing your children to make decisions, having rules in place and showing your affection.

When children turn two, they will start to understand the process of discipline. Make sure they know the rules of the house and that you both stay consistent. Children will start to know which parent is more lenient, who caves, and they will start to use it to their advantage. This is a time of testing the discipline...you are the teacher and they are the student.

How children Learn - Respect their Individuality

As parents, we hook the attention and put information in their minds through repetition. This is the way we learn everything we know. As children we learn how to behave in society, what to believe and not believe, what is acceptable and not, good, bad, beautiful, ugly, right and wrong. In school we put attention on what the teacher is teaching, in church what the preacher is preaching, and at home, discipline from the parents. This attention from others develops into a need for attention and we become competitive. "Look at what I am doing". Children are a product of their parents; they don't get to pick their name, religion, language, morals or values. Children just agree with the information being passed on to them. When children agree with it, they believe it and this is what we call faith, to believe unconditionally. Children believe everything adults say.

Some children are domesticated the same way we domesticate a dog. In order to teach the dog we punish the dog when bad and reward the dog when good. We teach our children the same way. We tell them good boy or good girl when they do what parents ask if them; and when they go against the rules, they are punished. Soon they become afraid of being punished and afraid of not receiving the reward. The reward is the attention they get from their parents and teachers. They soon develop a need for reward and attention. They start becoming actors, pretending to be what we want them to be, not what they want to be. They are afraid of rejection, not being good enough or not pleasing others. They become a copy of their parents, teachers, church and television.

Effective and positive discipline is about teaching and guiding children, not just forcing them to obey. Discipline is the structure that helps the child fit into the real world happily and effectively. It is the foundation for the development of the child's own self-discipline. It is important to let our children learn things independently and make decisions early in life. Parenting is the task of raising children and providing them with all the necessary emotional support to further their physical, emotional, cognitive, spiritual and social development.

Late toddlers - 2 to 3 years

Toddlers continue to struggle with independence and self-control. They realize their limitations and can become frustrated when they cannot achieve a task. They also push for more independence and when they do not get their way, have temper tantrums. It is important to find out the meaning of their outbursts first and try to work through them with patience and empathy. It is also important to continue to set limits, keep routines and follow rules so they can continue to learn. Children respect and feel more comfortable when parents are in charge, knowing they are being protected. At this age, you can start to reason and explain to the child. When your child throws a tantrum, hold the child until they gain control. Then give the child a short explanation of why they cannot do this and redirect them to an activity. Continue with the process, but stay firm showing them you are in charge and they will not continue that behavior.

Preschoolers and kindergarten-age children – 3 to 5 years old

This is the stage where most children seek approval and praise. They love to hear they did a good job when helping with a chore or drawing a picture. They are able to begin to understand rules and how to follow them. They start to model behaviors, either good or bad, developing patterns from either one parent or a combo of both. For those of you who have been enforcing the rules, this age will be much easier because the child knows who the boss is. They have already worked out the majority of issues and you will only have occasional flair ups. For those of you who have not set limits, rules and roles, this can be a difficult time trying to establish discipline later in their lives.

Children will have different behavior routines for example if the daycare/school has instilled rules that the child has followed for years, they will continue with good behavior and follow the rules they are used to. If at home the rules are very slack, the child will act out with the bad behaviors and continue what they have learned at home.

Here is where verbal rules and directions start to increase. Parents and schools may start to use short time outs when they misbehave. If your child gets up, you will need to re-direct them back to the chair a few times and verbally tell them why. You can sit with them at first with a clock and show them how much time they have left. As they get used to this, you will tell them they have 2 minutes and sit near them. You can continue to move further apart and increase time as needed. Long lectures are not productive for children, as they do not understand what is going on.

A great way to help teach children good behaviors is a three-part process

1. Explain why
2. Take something away
3. Have them help to correct the situation

Always use patience and a calm voice when using discipline. It is important to use reason when teaching children right from wrong.

1. If a child throws food on the floor
    a. Explain to him/her this is wasting food
    b. Show them how much money they are wasting; take 25 cents from their bank
    c. Have them clean the floor because they made it dirty

2. If your child paints on your table
    a. Explain why it destroys the table
    b. Take their paints away for a day
    c. Have them clean up the table

3. If your child breaks a toy
    a. Have them to explain why they broke a toy
    b. Have them throw away the toy
    c. Take money from their bank showing they wasted money

School-age children (6 years to 8 years)

Children are starting to choose their friends, the activities they enjoy and starting to become very self-reliant. Many parents are so used to disciplining that they do not recognize this new independence. They try to control their kids, not letting them figure some things out on their own. Parents need to continue to supervise, model good behavior and set rules to follow, but at the same time, they need to observe and appreciate their autonomy. This is a good time to encourage and involve their kids to make small decisions on their own.

This could mean picking out what clothes they want to wear, what they want for dinner, what movie they would like to watch. Continue to praise, approve and show admiration generously for your children's accomplishments. Example: they did a great job in soccer today or got an A on a spelling test.

Adolescents

Conflicts will happen when your adolescent wants to individuate and may challenge family values and rules. Kids will become more influenced because of peer groups, and may start to distance themselves from parents. Parents can meet these challenges by remaining available, setting rules in a noncritical way, not belittling the adolescent, and avoiding lectures or predicting catastrophes. Contracting with the adolescent is also a useful tool. This can be very helpful by writing down the problem on paper, letting them help with the disciplined action, and signing their name to it. Disciplinary spanking of adolescents is most inappropriate and will cause anger and more distance.

Despite their challenging attitudes and professions of independence, many adolescents do want parental guidance and approval. Parents should ensure that the basic rules are followed and that logical consequences are set and kept in a non-confrontational way.

Positive Disciplining For All Ages

1. Look for good behavior and praise your kids.
2. Start early when you kids are babies to make it easy for you and your child.
3. Be consistent with your rules; kids love a routine.
4. Sit down calmly to explain behaviors, act out solutions with little kids, and let bigger kids be involved in the process of consequences.
5. Be particular with what really needs correction or punishment (don't sweat the small stuff).
6. Do not make threats of punishment that you do not carry through. This can be the biggest mistake parents make and just encourages kids to misbehave. You are sending a message of maybe I will and maybe

I won't. So each time, kids will go through the agonizing process of pushing the limits.

7. Set reasonable punishments. Little kids need a few minutes in a time out where older kids may need their phones taken away, or a weekend on restriction. Don't be unrealistic by using more than a few days of punishment…it just doesn't work.
8. Pick and choose your battles; always go for safety first, with all ages. Focus on what is really important. For small children only pick a few a day to work on.
9. Accidents will happen…at all ages. Do not punish for things that definitely are accidents. Know the difference between on purpose and accidentally. If you child spills their water once have them help clean it up, but tell them it was by accident. If they do it every night to get a laugh or negative attention, put them in a time out. Next day sit next to them and monitor the water.
10. Use positive rewards: gold stars, a special TV show or movie, some popcorn, and extra book.
11. Do not argue with your child. Just stay positive and repeat what you are saying.
12. Other acceptable means of discipline include withdrawal or delay of privileges such as TV, movies, games, etc.

"Feelings…Nothing more than feelings"

It is so important for your child to be able to identify how they are feeling. It is easier for young kids to point to a picture to identify their feelings. Go to the **Muppet Feelings Chart at pinterest.com/pin/2814818492644657**. It is important to educate your children that these are feelings, not who they are. Example: Kids have bad behavior they are not bad. Behaviors can be changed.

Always use I statements not you Statements

a. "You are lazy and did not pick up your toys like I told you" NO NO
b. "I do feel sad (feeling) when the toys are not picked up, it makes me feel messy when your room is messy" YES YES

a. "You are so stupid...you never finish your homework"
b. "I am really disappointed (feeling) when I learn your homework wasn't done." YES YES

Which is the best way to deliver consequences?

The best way to deliver consequences is with love. You kids will appreciate an explanation telling them **what** they did, **when** they did and **how** they did. You can ask them **why** they did it and have them identify the feeling associated with the act. Make sure you explain that the consequence is for bad behavior (punishing because of the act); explain that they are not a bad person (not punishing the person.) NEVER yell, humiliate, put down, shout obscenities, or bring up past mistakes, even if they are repeating the same behavior.

Three ways to discipline - Reasoning, Distraction and Discussion

Discipline involves teaching positive behavior so children are clear and will know what to do; what is good behavior. Parents also need to change unwanted behavior and teach them what not to do. *Distracting* young children away from the bad behavior is the best way to start discipline and keep them safe. *Reasoning* is effective for older children when they are old enough to understand, usually around 3 years of age. For children older than three, having a *Discussion* and teaching children desirable behaviors in advance is a great way to prevent the bad behavior. It is always better to prevent a behavior than to have to punish a child for the behavior. With all discipline, it is important to refrain from putting the child down or hurting their feelings. Self-esteem is the most important development for our children. We want them to individuate and have a healthy opinion about themselves. This in turn helps them to have healthy relationship with parents, siblings, friends and teachers.

Time-Out

Time-Out is one of the most effective disciplinary techniques available to parents of young children, aged two years through 5 years. This works well because the child receives a direct message that the behavior they are being punished for is inappropriate. It must be used consistently every time your child misbehaves to be effective, but not more than three times in a day. Time-outs can be very effective and when used properly they will to decrease in frequency.

Using a count of 1,2, 3, is a great way to help decrease the time-outs. This gives your child time to change their behavior to avoid the punishment. If the child does not change by the count of 3, you must continue with the time-out.

Here are some helpful hints for the most successful time-outs

1. Start your time-outs by 24 months.
2. Choose a place in your home where they will not be able to see television or play with any of their toys.
3. The best time for a time-out is 1 minute per year of age, not to exceed 5 minutes. You may have to start with 30 seconds at the beginning.
4. Use a timer and make sure you keep track. You can show your child the time so they can watch the time limit.
5. You can prepare your child by letting them know why they are in time-out. Use a very short sentence such as: no throwing your food, no biting, no hitting.
6. You will need to avoid talking to your child, meaning you will have to ignore them during this time. Even if they cry or yell you will need to let them express themselves. This has to happen so they know the meaning of time-out or this will not work. If they get up, you will need to walk them back over. You can redirect them three times only but make sure you do not make eye contact or talk to them. After that, the session is over. Start fresh the next time you have a behavior issue. Hang in there…be strong…know this is what is best for you and your child.
7. After the time-out, it is best to start fresh on a new activity, give them some affection.

What's Wrong with a Little Swat or Spanking

Some parents think it is okay to swat a kid on the hand or the bottom. Many of us got spankings with a belt or parent's hand and we turned out ok. As your child grows, that little swat will not be enough to stop behaviors, so you will have to have to use more strength. The reason behind a whipping is to instill fear so that the threat of a spanking will stop the behavior. Children mimic what they learn from us, so they may start to hit children in school thinking it is acceptable behavior. In addition, some children grow up with aggression and may abuse people closest to them. Spanking teaches an inner sense of wrong and that hitting is a way to deal with frustration. When parents become out of control themselves, this is when physical harm to a child can be dangerous.

The Psychosocial Pediatrics Committee of the Canadian Pediatric Society has carefully reviewed the available research in the controversial area of disciplinary spanking and supports the position that spanking and other forms of physical punishment are associated with negative child outcomes. The Canadian Pediatric Society strongly discourages disciplinary spanking and all other forms of physical punishment. Physical redirection or restraint to support time-out or to prevent a child from harming himself or others may be necessary, but should be done carefully and without violence.

13

"AND ON THIS FARM HE HAD A COW" BREASTFEEDING, FORMULA, MILK

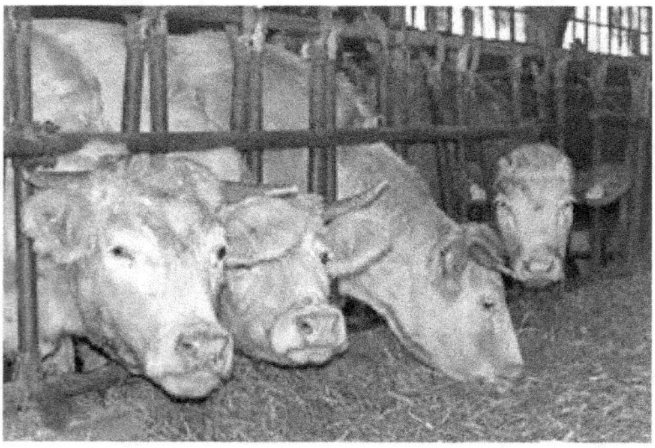

This is not how farm animals should be treated, but the truth is, this is how most non-organic cows are raised. It makes me sick to my stomach to see how these precious animals are caged inside without sunlight. I am not condemning meat, but I ask everyone to buy their meat from an organic farm, where the animals are allowed to see the light of day, feed on grass and walk around on God's great earth. What a cruel life; to stand or lie in a cage where they cannot even turn around. This also pertains to chickens, turkeys, calves, and pigs.

A Mother Cow Cries for Her Baby

Did you know that calves are taken from their moms as soon as they are born? The relationship and bond between a mother and her calf is immediate. Both the mom and their calves show emotional distress upon separation. They are not allowed to nurse their young just so humans can consume milk. The calves are given a powdered milk substitute. When mother cows are separated from their babies, they can be heard bellowing, a very loud cry, for days to weeks, showing they are suffering great emotional distress from their separation. It has also been shown that they will hover near a pen door where they last saw their calf. The calves have been known to try and suckle human fingers and form relationships with farmers and their helpers. The female calves will be raised to become milking cows like their mommies. Remember, the only way we get milk is from a pregnant, lactating cow. However, the male calves will go to be slaughtered and will continue to suffer by being placed in cages to keep them from developing muscles; this meat is called veal and is very tender.

If you are in need of a good cry watch this YouTube video.
https://www.youtube.com/watch?v=SYJPbrxdn8w

"Milk Does Not Do a Body Good"

None of us wants to hear this but dairy is one of the most inflammatory foods in our diet. Hot, gooey, melted cheese is most delicious but is on the "naughty" list. Many of us are not aware of it, but most of the population cannot handle dairy. It causes inflammation resulting in digestive issues such as gas, bloating, constipation, and diarrhea. Some people are lactose intolerant; they have problems with the sugar found in milk. Others have problems with protein, the casein and whey. Casein has a molecular structure close to gluten. If that is not enough, know that if you are not drinking organic milk, you are consuming a mixed cocktail of chemicals, antibiotics and growth hormones.

Dairy Products to Avoid

- Butter and butter fat
- Cheese
- Cottage cheese
- Cream
- Sour cream and cream cheese
- All milk, including buttermilk, powdered milk, and evaporated milk
- All yogurt including Greek
- Ice cream
- Pudding

Butter

Butter has hydrogen peroxide as a bleaching agent, yellow No. 3 coloring and nordihydroguaiaretic acid as an antioxidant. Again...Buy Organic!

"Wipe off that Mustache" - Dangers of Milk

Non-organic milk contains hydrogen peroxide, oat gum, antibiotics, fungicides, pesticides and hormones. In addition to milk, make sure if you must use dairy, purchase all of your cheese, cottage cheese, yogurt and all other dairy under the organic label. When buying cheese, consider purchasing a hard cheese that has been aged at least 6 months and organic. Buy Organic!

I imagine many adults and children are consuming more than 50% of their diets eating non-organic meats, milk and cheese. At what point do we call this safe consumption, when ingesting such high levels of hormones while eating high amounts of daily protein? The more non-organic dairy we eat, the more chemicals we ingest. The following is a study relating to hormone cancers and dairy.

Ganmaa Davaasambuu is a physician (Mongolia), a Ph.D. in environmental health (Japan), and a working scientist (Harvard School of Public Health). Her studies have led her to be suspicious in the role cow milk, cheese and other dairy products play in the hormone cancers including prostate, testes and breast. "The link between cancer and dietary hormones, estrogen in particular, has been a source of great concern among scientists", said Ganmaa, "but it has not been widely studied or discussed". She feels the potential risk is large. "Natural estrogens are up to 100,000 times more potent than their environmental counterparts, such as the estrogen-like compounds in pesticides".

Ganmaa is quoted as saying, "Among the routes of human exposure to estrogens, we are mostly concerned about cow's milk, which contains considerable amounts of female sex hormones. Part of the problem seems to be milk from modern dairy farms where cows are milked about 300 days a year. For much of that time, the cows are pregnant. The later in pregnancy a cow is the more hormones appear in her milk. **Milk from a cow in the late stage of pregnancy contains up to 33 times as much of a signature estrogen compound** (estrone sulfate) than milk from a non-pregnant cow and 10 times more progesterone than raw."

According to Ganmaa, "butter, meat, eggs, milk, and cheese are implicated in higher rates of hormone-dependent cancers in general". Furthermore, "breast cancer has been linked particularly to consumption of milk and cheese. In another study, rats fed milk show a higher incidence of cancer and develop a higher number of tumors than those who drank water".

Many doctors, commercials or surveys will try to convince us that if our children do not use milk their bones will not develop. The following chart shows that there are **much healthier ways to get our calcium**.

Bok Choy	222 mg	3	cup
Collard greens	360 mg	3.5	cups
Kale	300 mg	3	cups
Tofu	434 mg	½	cup
Milk	305 mg	1	cup (**Not recommended**)
Broccoli	129 mg	3	cups
Sesame seeds	264 mg	3	tbsp

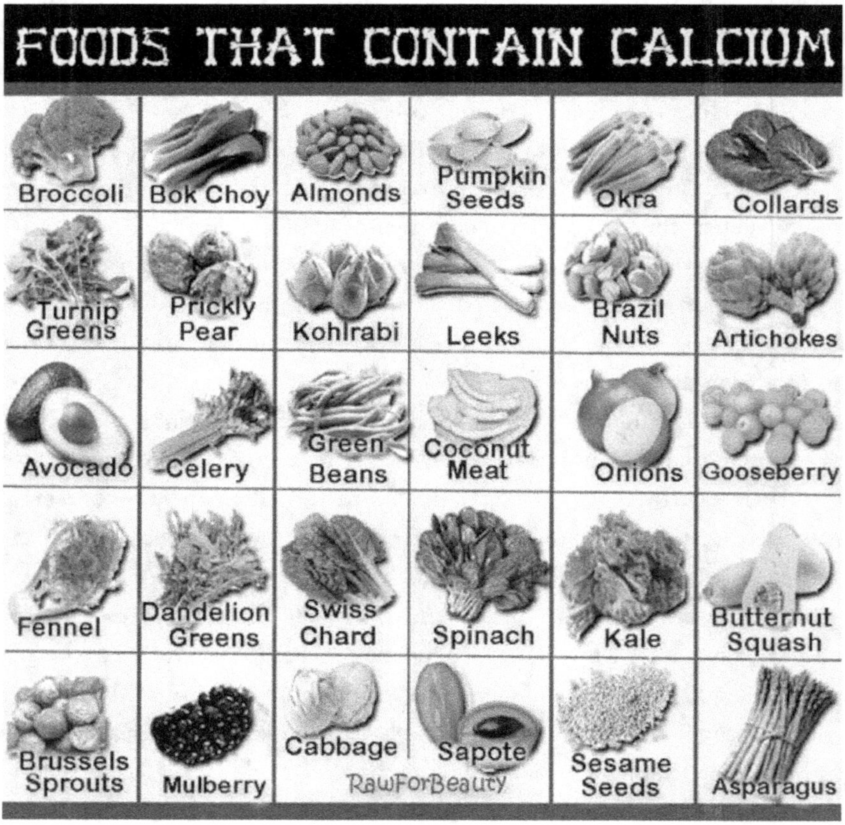

Dangers for Using Infant Formula

Infant formula is a manufactured, processed, mostly GMO, non-organic combination of chemicals concocted to mimic breast milk. Infant formula is an 8 billion dollars a year business. There is a large variety of different brands of infant formulas available and a wide range of specialty formulas available for babies with problems associated with prematurity, lactose intolerance, milk allergy, reflux and other serious conditions/disorders. It is fast and convenient and many parents use it exclusively or in a pinch when in a hurry. Some mothers go back to work early and find the pumping inconvenient. Let us look at some statistics that will hopefully steer you away from processed infant formula. Breast milk is the best choice and has superior nutrients including 160 fatty acids that your baby needs. Even if you are going back to work in six weeks, it is still a huge benefit to breast feed your babies to give them a healthy start in life.

Canned Liquid Formula

When using liquid formula, you need to be aware that most cans contain the toxic chemical BPA. We already know of its use in plastic but it is in the lining of the metal cans too. The BPA is supposed to protect the food from directly contacting the metal. When food is exposed to the BPA, even small amounts may migrate into the liquid or food.

"But testing by EWG and by the Food and Drug Administration (FDA) indicates that under normal use, liquid formula itself could expose an infant to substantially more BPA than a plastic bottle. An August 2007 investigation by EWG estimated that at BPA levels found in ready-to-eat liquid formula, 1 of every 16 infants fed the formula would be exposed to the chemical at doses exceeding those that caused harm in laboratory studies."

What are These Products Doing in Canned and Powdered Formula?

Cupric Sulfate (Copper Sulfate)

A compound combines sulfur with copper. It is a pesticide, herbicide and fungicide that kills bacteria, plants, algae, snails, and fungi. It can be found in foods, water and the environment and is classified as an irritant, dangerous to the environment, and exposure can lead to many health problems. It has registered for use in pesticides in the U.S. since 1956.

Polydextrose

The FDA approved Polydextrose in 1981 as a food ingredient synthesized from dextrose (glucose). It is a newfangled soluble fiber additive which is being added to dairy, baked goods, and you guessed it, infant formula. It is primarily used to increase fiber, replace sugar, and to reduce fat and calories. It bulks up reduced-calorie products and makes them taste better, while showing more fiber on the food label.

Nonfat Milk

The most common infant formulas consumed by infants are made from modified cow's milk with added carbohydrate (usually lactose), vegetable oils, and vitamins and minerals. Nonfat milk is the first ingredient on the list and in a powdered form, can be preserved for many months without spoiling. Unless it is labeled organic, it will have hormones and antibiotics, which are not recommended at any age for your child.

Soy Oil

Soybeans are legumes that originated in East Asia, but are now being produced on a large scale in the United States. Soy is very inexpensive and is used in tofu, soy milk and various dairy and meat substitutes. The problem with soybean oil is that it is a trans fat and the worst kind of fat available. Partial hydrogenation is the process that turns good oil into bad oil. This process makes the oil more solid and gives a longer shelf life. Over 90% of soy produced in the U.S. is genetically modified. The problem with GMO's is that the crops are engineered to be herbicide tolerant which means farmers need to use more toxic herbicides. Crops that are sprayed with the herbicide Roundup have been linked with adverse health effects like sterility, birth defects, cancer and hormone problems. Soybean oil is extracted from soybean seeds and are also used as a base in paints and printer ink, because it hardens when exposed to air.

Lactose

Lactase is an enzyme, or chemical, the sugar or carbohydrate found in milk, which the body uses to digest the sugar in milk (lactose). Lactose is the milk produced in the breast by all mammals but is not found anywhere else in nature. The amount of lactose in breast milk varies depending on a mother's consumption of lactose and averages between 7% and 9%. Cow's milk contains approximately 4.7%. Most infant formulas contain a similar percentage of lactose as breast milk.

More and more babies are lactose intolerant today. This means there is not enough lactase or undigested milk sugar and when it gets into the large bowel, it causes gut pains and diarrhea. If your child were colicky, this would be an area to explore. Many people substitute a soy-based formula, which contains no lactose, however, many babies are allergic to soy products also.

"Eating Your Curds & Whey" - Whey Protein Concentrate

Whey protein is the watery portion of milk that separates from the curds when making cheese. Whey protein is our building blocks called amino acids, which primarily are used for muscle growth and to repair tissues. There is a higher percentage of whey protein found in breast milk (60%), compared to cow's milk (20%). Formula companies try to mimic the amount of whey protein found in breast milk by using whey protein concentrate. It is processed and homogenized, eliminating most of the nutrients and making it the least expensive form of whey protein.

High Oleic Safflower Oil

This ingredient is used in processed food. The reason why manufacturers use high oleic safflower oil is to extend the shelf life of their products.

Powdered Infant Formula

Infant formula that is made with powdered ingredients can be the most toxic of all, because it is mixed with our own water source. Many of us do not have a proper filtration system installed in our homes. A filtration system is needed if you have well water or municipal/city water. We already know not to use a BPA container filled with water because of the chemicals that have leeched into the water. Our water can contain bacteria, chlorine byproducts, pesticides, lead, solvents, arsenic or nitrates from fertilizer runoff. If you must use a prepared infant formula, use the organic powdered formula with water from either a BPA free container or install a water conditioning system under your kitchen sink.

Perchlorate

"And Bingo"...There is yet another reason to be cautious about using powdered infant formula and "it's name-O" is perchlorate. Perchlorate is found in typical groundwater and surface water conditions and originates from disinfectants, bleaching agents, herbicides, and mostly from rocket propellant runoffs into the ground. High levels of perchlorate affect the thyroid gland by blocking its ability to use iodine. The thyroid produces a hormone that is essential for proper brain development of fetuses and infants. "CDC studies have shown that nearly everyone in the U.S. is exposed regularly to low levels of perchlorate. People are exposed through eating food, and drinking milk and water that contain perchlorate. Trace levels of perchlorate have been found in both breast milk and infant formula."

The federal Centers for Disease Control and Prevention (CDC) have found perchlorate in powdered infant formula. The study found that two most contaminated brands, made from cow's milk, accounted for 87 percent of the U.S. powdered formula market in 2000. They purchased three different samples of five different brands after visiting five different stores. Two widely distributed different brands of bovine milk-based with lactose had significantly higher perchlorate levels than all of the other bovine milk-based with lactose. All of the powdered infant formulas tested contained perchlorate. Cow's milk-based formula with lactose had a significantly higher concentration of perchlorate than the other types.

The CDC's recent study of perchlorate in infant formula published in *The Journal of Exposure Science and Environmental Epidemiology 1.*

Check Off List to Prepare Formula

1. If you must prepare formula, make sure to wash your hands first, and clean the counter space.
2. Always sterilize bottles, nipples, caps and rings before daily use and especially right out of the container. Sterilize by boiling all pieces in good quality water for at least 5-7 minutes.
3. If buying prepared formula, make sure to buy organic. Check the expiration dates and make sure the can is not damaged
4. Shake formula before using and follow directions on the can exactly.
5. Wash the outside of the can/lid (bacteria can live on the lid).
6. Warm the formula by placing the bottle in hot water, NOT BOILING, or run under warm water for a few minutes.
7. Make sure your bottles and all accessories are BPA free.
8. Be sure to smell the canned formula, check for discolored or curdled formula.
9. Check with your doctor if you can use organic powdered formula especially for premature babies, babies under two months, or those who have a compromised immune system.
10. For powdered formula, use filtered water and let it run a few minutes first to reduce contaminants.
11. Never warm a bottle in the microwave.
12. Follow directions on cans and do not to exceed expiration dates for open cans.
13. Formula is best used fresh and not kept out in room temperature

"There's A Hole in My Bucket"

Women and Men need to drink an adequate amount of water. It is best to drink your own water from home. You may want to obtain a municipal water report, testing for lead, mercury, nitrates, E-coli and bacteria. This report is yours by law and most states offer the test at a very inexpensive price or free.

Choices for Safer Water

- The most inexpensive would be to use one a drip water filter systems that filters into a pitcher.
- A step up is to install a filter system under your kitchen sink to use for drinking water.
- You will also need to add a filtered shower nozzle. Many people do not realize that when you jump into a warm shower you are opening up your pores and allowing all of those chemicals to enter and contaminate your body.
- For those fortunate families, it is best to install a whole house system. Below is a very affordable system from Premier Research Labs.

Keep you and your family safe with a reverse osmosis filtration system

Reverse osmosis filtration system - for clean and healthy drinking water. Our bodies are made up of 55-60% water, and drinking healthy, purified water is crucial to living a happy and energetic life. I use a system from Premier Research Labs, which is very inexpensive. It is designed to fit underneath your sink, so it is out of sight but never out of mind. I also use premiers shower filter nozzles. These are a very inexpensive way to protect your family.

Shower Head - Premier's shower head has a filter that converts chlorine into a harmless soluble chloride for better lathering with healthier water. Without a filter a hot shower turns the chlorine into a gaseous vapor that contaminates our skin, as well as our respiratory system, kidneys, and various other organs in our bodies. This shower head is in most people's budget.

The good news is that everywhere you go these days; you see people drinking water. However, the majority are carrying water in toxic water bottles. The problem with bottled water is twofold; the quality of the water in the bottle and the plastic bottle itself. Unless a bottle is marked BPA free, it contains the toxins BPA. BPA stands for bisphenol A. BPA is an industrial chemical that has been used to make certain plastics and resins since the 1960's. BPA is found in polycarbonate plastics and epoxy resins. Polycarbonate plastics are often used in containers that store food and beverages, such as water bottles and metal cans. Some research has shown that BPA can seep into food or beverages from containers that are made with BPA. There are some health concerns with **BPA having negative effects on the brain, behavior and prostate gland of fetuses, infants and children.**

The Food and Drug Administration (FDA) has stated that BPA is safe at the very low levels that occur in some foods. However, at the same time gives the following suggestions from their website:

Here is information for consumers who want to limit their exposure to BPA:

- Plastic containers have recycle codes on the bottom. Some, but not all, plastics that are marked with recycle codes 3 or 7 may be made with BPA.

- Do not put very hot or boiling liquid that you intend to consume in plastic containers made with BPA. BPA levels rise in food when containers/products made with the chemical are heated and come in contact with the food
- Discard all bottles with scratches as they may harbor bacteria and have a greater chance of releasing BPA.

They openly admit not to put hot liquids into plastic made with BPA. Another thing to consider is to never buy your bottled water where it is sitting out in the hot sun. Have you ever driven up to a gas station and see cases of water just sitting out in the sun heating up the chemicals inside?

Buy Glass! Glass is your best option or purchase BPA free plastic containers. They are clearly marked on the bottles.

How Much Water Should We Drink?

Every system in your body needs water. Water is one way to flush the toxins out of the organs. It also carries nutrients to your cells. We lose water through urine, bowel movements and perspiration. It is best to consume 1/2 ounce of water for every pound of weight. Some have made estimates that men need about 12 cups (96 ounces) a day where women need about 8 cups (64 ounces) a day. If you are drinking herbal hot or cold tea beverages with no additives such as sugar, this can be counted as part of your water consumption.

Got Milk? Yes Mommies Milk Please

The safest choice is clear: Breast feed your baby whenever possible. Breast milk is the best source of nutrition for babies. It contains essential fatty acids that help bolster babies' bodies against the impacts of toxic chemicals. However, there are many reasons why families rely on formula for some or all of their baby's diet. Seventy percent of babies in the U.S. receive some formula by the time they are 3 months old. These babies need a safe and healthy source of food, and formula should be manufactured in a way that avoids contamination with harmful chemicals.

14

"DO YOU KNOW THE MUFFIN MAN?" WHITE FLOUR & SUGAR

It's nine am and we walk by the Cinnabon bakery? The smell is so delightful; so how do we fight temptation. Do we want to satisfy a quick craving and jeopardize our health? Well, let us see; it has sugar and white flour, everything we need for a fast blast of pleasure. If you are used to eating this way, it is hard to give up this lifestyle. This is how so many people wake up every day because it is quick, convenient and tastes delicious. We add a large coffee and we are off to the races. This is the fastest way to gain weight and load our body with toxins by consuming simple carbohydrates, which are not only very tasty but also very addictive. When you eat carbs, your blood sugar rapidly rises. You get a temporary "high" when your blood sugar is high. Next, a blast of insulin from the pancreas causes a drop in blood sugar. At this point, feelings of weakness, fatigue, shakiness and even anxiety can set in. In order to feel good again, a person will indulge by eating another blast of carbs. This vicious cycle is exactly what happens to drug addicts/alcoholics, who must continue to have repeated "fixes" of their drug in order to feel good.

Cancer cells are also fueled by and live on carbs and sugar. Remember that simple carbs act exactly like a sugar in the body.

Besides, we all know that carbs are our comfort food. Carbs increase brain levels of tryptophan, which is the amino acid that converts to serotonin in the brain. Overeating carbs, including breads, pastas, chips, and cookies, can temporarily help with depression, anxiety, and stress, giving us the instant lift we need. Most of us "self-medicate" due to cravings for these unhealthy carbs and sugars, which leads to unhealthy weight gain and disease.

A high-carb diet rich in simple carbohydrates, including starches/breads, will cause you to gain weight, which can contribute to insulin resistance and Diabetes 2. When the blood glucose is too high, the pancreas becomes overworked trying to produce enough insulin to compensate for the high blood glucose. Type 2 Diabetes occurs when there is too much fat on the blood cells and the pancreas does not produce enough insulin.

According to the American Diabetes Association, carbohydrates include the following three: **Complex carbohydrates (starches), simple carbohydrates (sugars), and fibers.**

Complex carbs/starches (limit these); not all Carbs are created equal. The good part about complex carbs are that they digest slowly, prolong energy, are higher in fiber, and make us feel fuller longer. These carbs enter the bloodstream slower and trigger only a moderate rise in insulin levels and help to have fewer carbs to be stored as fat. The bad complex carbohydrates include peas, corn, lima beans, white potatoes, and all grains including wheat, oats, pasta, corn, etc. However, the carbs listed below should be limited or eliminated for those who are having trouble losing weight and are ill with disease, disorders or food intolerances/allergies.

Complex Carbs - so *"a little dab 'll do ya"*

- Bagels
- Baked beans
- Buckwheat
- Cakes
- Candy
- Cereals
- Cookies
- Corn
- Cornmeal
- Crackers
- High fiber cereals
- Jam
- Juice
- Macaroni
- Pastas
- Peas
- Pita bread
- White potatoes
- White rice
- Soda
- Soy milk
- Soybeans
- Spaghetti
- Whole barley
- Whole grain flours
- Whole meal bread

Better Choices

- Sweet potatoes
- Whole grain products
- Wild, brown, or black rice
- Multi grain bread
- Oat bran
- Oatmeal
- All beans

White Foods / Black list

The truth about white foods, they are "the bad carbs": white flour, white rice, white sugar and white salt. That means all pre-packaged junk food like cookies, cakes, candies and pretzels are all on the bad list. Therefore, you need to kiss white foods goodbye if you want to stay healthy, keep your kids healthy, lose weight and heal illness. So what is all the hubbub about?

"White, Don't Bite It" White Flour

Bread, the "slice of life" just does not stack up in the health industry. What is the difference between white bread and whole grain? Once the bread is stripped of the bran, the germ layers have been removed and the flour is bleached with chemicals such as potassium bromate or chlorine dioxide, you are left with a starch. Starch and Sugar are one in the same; they put you on a roller coaster high, only to crash and burn later. Then the cravings start and you want more and more. While white bread is so soft and light, and melts in your mouth, there are no nutrients in white bread products. The slogan should have been "helps tear down your body 12 ways." I know we could all just live and breathe bread and butter, not to mention its nurturing abilities.

So you don't "knead the bread spread or the leaven rise" going straight to your butt or thighs, so leave the following alone:

- White bread
- White pasta
- White wraps
- White rice
- White pizza crust
- White rolls
- White muffins
- White baked goods
- White bagels

Gluten Free Breads

Gluten free foods, breads, pastas and pastries, are a multibillion-dollar industry and can be purchased in many restaurants and supermarkets. Gluten is the protein that is found in grains such as wheat, spelt, barley, oats and rye. Many people are gluten intolerant, have leaky gut syndrome, or celiac disease, where inflammation interferes with digestion. Gluten free does not necessarily mean healthy, meaning corn and rice can have damaging inflammatory effects on the body. Quinoa and amaranth also carry the label, and are an excellent healthier choice. Soy is a cheap grain and is genetically modified (GMO) and contains phytoestrogens which can wreak havoc on our bodies. The major problem with most gluten free products is that they contain refined sugar and unhealthy vegetable oils. "*Bake the Very Best*" Quinoa and amaranth are an excellent healthier choice and organic grain-free flour alternatives such as coconut, hazelnut and almond flours. These are my favorites and they contain protein and hardly any carbs. If you have a nut allergy, you will need to stay away from these.

"Rice a Phony" White Rice

____Not such a treat! When rice is harvested, it first has the husk removed, which leaves brown rice. Then the bran layer and germ are removed, along with the vitamins and minerals, making it white rice. Then a glucose layer is added to make it shine. It is not hair, just saying. If a product says enriched, it means quite the opposite. It is not "rich" it is actually a "poor" quality food; it has been robbed of its nutrients.

In the last ten years, scientists have found high levels of arsenic in rice. Rice plants have the ability to absorb toxins from the soil more than any other grain. Arsenic has also been found in beer, when rice is used as an ingredient. It has been found in rice beverages when used as a replacement for milk. Also, beware of brown rice syrup, which is an additive in many products. Arsenic is an element in the Earth's crust and is present in very small amounts in water, soil and air. Crops absorb arsenic as they grow. That is how it gets into foods and beverages — it is not an additive or ingredient — and it cannot be completely eliminated.

Arsenic in rice - limit in Pregnancy & Infants

In 2013, FDA released test data from 1300 samples of rice and rice product levels of inorganic arsenic in the US. The test included infant rice cereal since they consume three times more than adults and at 8 months is the centerpiece of their diet. Arsenic is a carcinogen, an increased chance of developing cancer (lung and bladder) and the FDA has a body of scientific studies linking compromised pregnancy outcomes with high intakes of the rice. In addition, children have shown decreased performance with developmental tests that measure learning. The FDA is proposing a limit or 100 parts per billion of arsenic in infant rice cereals. The FDA is asking food manufacturers to reduce the limits and when testing 76 samples, half of them meet the limits. However, the other half do not. Buy organic brands, make sure to use other infant cereals including oats, quinoa and amaranth.

Make your Brown Rice like Pasta

The Dr. Oz show recently aired a segment showing the new recommendations from the FDA regarding arsenic in rice. The safest types of rice to buy is Basmati rice which is produced in California, Pakistan and India, or sushi rice. These tested a much lower arsenic level.

Tip: Boil your rice like pasta. For every one cup of rice, add 6 cups of water. Cook until done. Pour off excess water through a strainer to remove as much of the arsenic as possible. Puree and store in the refrigerator.

Simple Carbohydrates/Sugar

In the 1800's people consumed about 18 pounds of sugar a year, in the 1900's 90 pounds of sugar, and in **2009, 180 pounds of sugar**. Sugar is in everything: soft drinks, fruit drinks, sauces, processed foods, canned foods, and you will not believe this one, most infant formula.....come on! Check for yourself; most infant formulas contain sugar or corn syrup. No wonder kids are addicted to sugar so early in life.

There are naturally occurring sugars in fruits or milk (lactose). There are added sugars such as table sugar added to a cookie or heavy syrup, which is added to canned fruit. There are so many different sugars such as table sugar, brown sugar, beet sugar, cane sugar, raw sugar, fruit sugar (fructose), turbinado, and high fructose corn syrup. Sounds like a song! Simple Sugars also include glucose (also known as dextrose), sucrose, fructose and galactose. The worst sugar is high fructose corn syrup, 55 percent fructose and 45 percent glucose. Simple carbs digest quickly, give a slow burst of energy, are low in fiber, make you hungry sooner and convert to fat cells.

High Fructose Corn Syrup (Stop Eating this or Gain Weight Fast)

Today, 55 percent of sweeteners used in food and beverage manufacturing are made from corn; and the number one source of calories in America's soda is, high fructose corn syrup. In the 1970's, food and beverage manufacturers began switching their sweeteners from sucrose to corn syrup…why? Wait for it…..MONEY. They found out the high fructose corn syrup was much cheaper. It is also much sweeter than table sugar so they could use less. It does not stop there; studies have shown that it can lead more specifically to belly fat gain. Other health risks include **elevated blood sugar, high blood pressure, elevated LDL (low-density lipoprotein), and decreased HDL (high-density lipoprotein), elevated triglycerides and non-alcoholic fatty liver disease, which is alcohol without the buzz.** It is time to eliminate high fructose corn syrup. Corn syrup tricks your body into gaining weight by fooling your metabolism. It turns off your body's appetite-control system, which results in an increased appetite to eat more. It does not appropriately stimulate insulin, which does not suppress the hunger hormone ghrelin. It also does not stimulate the satiety hormone leptin. So with this combination, you do not know when to stop eating and you do not feel full. And *"that's how the cookie crumbles."*

Sugar Alcohols

Sugar alcohols are used in sugar-free candies. They include sorbitol, maltitol, xylitol, glycerol, erythritol and mannitol. They do not absorb completely into the small intestine so they have fewer calories than sugar but are known to cause diarrhea, flatulence and bloating.

Artificial Sweeteners

Artificial sweeteners are not sugars. They are chlorinated sweeteners, and very toxic chemicals. The following artificial sweeteners approved by the FDA include acesulfame, aspartame, saccharin, sucralose, and neotame. They are added to many baked goods and diet drinks to reduce the calories. However, just because they are approved does not mean they are healthy for you. Sucralose/Splenda in the yellow pack was marketed as being made from sugar, however, it is the same as aspartame (the blue pack) and saccharin (the pink pack); it is just another chemical.

Michael G. Tordoff, Department of Neurobiology, Physiology and Behavior, University of California at Davis, has published several studies showing that artificial sweeteners can:

1. Increase hunger, short-term food intake, and cravings
2. Affect blood sugar levels, which can be especially dangerous to people with diabetes or epilepsy
3. Cause fluid retention
4. Increase cellulite
5. Contribute to weight gain

In one study, he found that the aspartame in chewing gum increased hunger due to oral stimulation by the added chemicals. His study also showed a gender-related sweetness response, which explains why certain people feel "ravenous" after consuming aspartame-containing products and others do not.

White Sugar

Simple carbs/white sugars are empty calories, have no nutritional value at all and are very dangerous carbs. When broken down and digested quickly, they leave you feeling tired, hungry, and craving more sugar shortly after you have eaten. Recent research has shown that certain simple carbohydrate foods can cause extreme surges in blood sugar levels, which also increases insulin release. This can elevate appetite and the risk of excess fat storage. Simply stay away from Simple Carbs! There are health risks that include the risk of obesity, diabetes, cardiovascular disease, gout in men and metabolic syndrome.

"Things Do Not go Better with Coke"

"Coke Adds Life". Are you kidding me? How far from the truth is this? Here is where some will draw the line, thinking there is no way they can give up their soda's and so called energy drinks. Soda pop, energy drinks, sports drinks and fruit juice are nothing more than heaping cups of chemicals. I am sorry to say but you *"can't have it your way"* here. They must go. I would like to recommend substituting your soda for a vitamin B supplement. I never leave the house without my B's and suggest ordering the Max B from Premier Research Labs. Have you ever really noticed a vitamin that really gave you energy? I have had more clients tell me that when they drink the B's they instantly have more energy without the sugar, corn syrup and caffeine. Watch out because most B's are made with coal tar. If your urine is bright yellow, discontinue the B supplement; this most likely means your supplement contains coal tar.

In the United States:

63 million people consume diet soda
158 million people consume sugar drinks

Wow! We can all agree that soda/drinks are high in calories, sugar, and low in nutrients. Soda contributes to obesity, tooth decay, weakens bones and starts caffeine dependence. Studies show that people have an unhealthy diet to go along with this. Many dentists call this the melting pot, as when you bathe your teeth in a citric acid and the sugar combo it breaks down the tissue, bone and teeth. I knew this at a very early age as I chewed about two packs of gum a day, back when gum came in a five pack. I had 16 cavities at one time, and had ten of those removed in the last two years.

Caffeine is a stimulant, that's right, like cocaine and tobacco, and it is considered a drug, which is why we become dependent on it. Have you ever tried to give up your cup of java? If so, you will notice detox/withdrawal symptoms: headaches, irritability, and a rise in blood pressure. Soda with sugar contains about 35 to 38 milligrams of caffeine per 12-ounce can. Diet soda packs in about 42 milligrams of caffeine. Diet soda is even a worse choice since the artificial sugar is a chemical and it contains more caffeine to boot.

Lose Energy with Energy Drinks

Most energy drinks claim to be a magic potion of vitamins and minerals to boost energy. Many have guarana, taurine, ginseng, and synthetic B vitamins made from coal tar. The manufacturers are not required to list whether the herbs have been sprayed with pesticides, or if they are synthetically made. Most sports and energy drinks contain the following: Sugar, Dextrose, Citric Acid, MSG, Natural Flavor, Salt, Sodium Citrate, Monopotassium, Phosphate, Gum Arabic, Sucrose, Acetate Isobutyrate, Glycerol, Ester of Rosin, and Yellow 6 dye.

Three ounces of sugar in any form such as fruit juice, soda, or sport drinks, suppresses the activity of white blood cells for up to 5 hours. It is estimated that Americans drink 22% of their total calories from beverages sweetened with sugar, high-fructose corn syrup, and artificial sweeteners.

"Good to the Last Drop" Coffee

Many people will agree that they love their coffee. Coffee contains caffeine, which artificially speeds up your body. You should be able to wake up and have energy on your own. Do you find that you need more and more coffee to make it through your day? "Don't be fooled that it is "mountain grown." Coffee is the heaviest chemically treated food in the world. Heavy synthetic nitrogen fertilizers are used when growing coffee. Human health concerns surrounding contamination include certain cancers, birth defects, blue baby syndrome, hypertension and developmental problems in children. Coffee is grown slowly in the rain forest, which like everything else in the world is too slow. So to speed up the process, 70 percent of the coffee bean is now grown in the sun as a resistant hybrid. Moldiness in green coffee may occur during curing, drying, and storage periods. Water damage of bagged coffee may also promote the growth of molds on the beans. The major pest attacking coffee beans is the coffee berry borer beetle. So make the "*best part of waking up*", Premier's B vitamins in your cup.

If you do want to consume coffee, make sure it is organic and limit yourself to one 8 oz. cup a day. Add cashew milk instead of cream, stevia or raw honey instead of sugar and enjoy your healthy cup of java.

White Salt

Iodized salt just may be the *"salt of the earth"*, but the better choice is Pink Sea Salt from the "salt of the sea." Almost every client I see will tell me they do not use salt because they think salt is unhealthy for them. They are right about table/white iodized salt because it is produced by taking natural tan colored salt (or crude oil flake leftovers) and heating it up to 1200° Fahrenheit; turning it into a white chemical.

What is so dangerous is that iodized salt is in nearly every prepackaged food we eat. Salt is used as a preservative, and on food items, it can kill living bacteria. Very few companies are using sea salt because of the expense and yes, *Greed!* Medical doctors will also insist that you do not use iodized salt because it can raise blood pressure very quickly since the blood is attempting to move toxins rapidly away from the heart. It also can be very damaging to the digestive system, cause dehydration as well as water retention; this can lead to increased problems for diabetes, gout and obesity.

The level of white salt in prepackaged foods is so high that over time it can cause destruction to major organs. Salt is also highly addictive, meaning the more you use, the more you want. This also leads us to a midnight snack, craving a salty snack such as potato chips and pretzels.

15

"I'M A LITTLE TEAPOT" - HEALTHY DRINKS FOR KIDS

Thirsty? Stay away from all processed drinks. This means no juice in jars, cans, boxes or plastic. Many have corn syrup or added sugar and even if they don't, they are processed and extremely high in sugar. See the quick and easy alternatives below to help you find a balance of delicious drinks for your kids:

 # 1 - Water: Water is essential for life; however, water should be offered AFTER THE AGE OF SIX MONTHS. Babies get their water from mommy's breast milk or formula. Water is not necessary under this age and could fill baby up so they do not want to nurse. It is the number one recommended drink after six months of age.

#2 - Homemade raw cold pressed juice: mostly vegetable juice made with a little fruit.

 # 3 - Homemade nut milk: Only takes 5 minutes to make!

<u>Ingredients</u>

1 cup raw almonds, walnuts or cashews soaked in filtered water
3 1/2 cups filtered water
1/4 teaspoon cinnamon
Small pinch of fine sea salt
2 soaked pitted dates (optional)
1/2 tsp vanilla extract

Directions

Soak 1 cup of selected nuts in water overnight (about 8-10 hours). Rinse and drain well. Add the nuts, cinnamon and sea salt to a blender with good quality filtered water. Blend for approximately 1 minute on high. Pour nut mixture over a nut milk bag or strainer. Refrigerate the milk and save the nuts for ingredients in other recipes. Use the milk for up to 3 days. Shake each time before using.

Store bought nut milk: Make sure you buy unsweetened almond, walnut, cashew, macadamia nut, coconut, hemp, etc. Avoid rice milks since they can contain higher levels of arsenic.

#4 – Smoothies – Homemade smoothies using nut milks, fruits and veggies. A wonderful tasty way to bring nourishment into your kids' lives.

#5 – Coconut Water – no sugar added

"Come Alive" Juicing

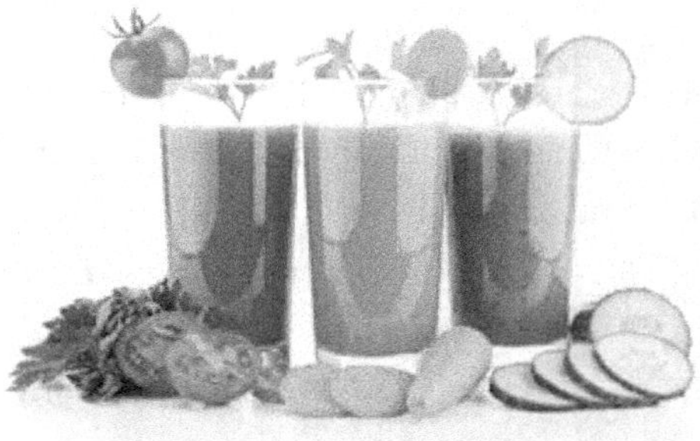

Juicing is one of the greatest drinks you can offer your kids - fresh, nutrient-dense, cold pressed homemade mostly vegetable juices. Juicing is a way to speed up your metabolism and immune system to help you heal from almost every major health challenge you have developed. Juicing places the body in a position to detoxify, allowing for pure antioxidants to boost the immune system.

65% of Americans are overweight or obese. Recent data out of John Hopkins University suggests this number will be 75% by 2015. One out of every three children born today will develop diabetes. Many of us are low in energy, suffer with chronic pain and a lack of focus. Our modern diet and lifestyle is to blame.

"If You're Green on the Inside, You're Clean on the Inside."

Homemade vegetable and fruit juice is low in calories, fat free, and nutrient dense. Fresh juice is very rich in vitamins, minerals, and antioxidants. It is a body boost, giving you and your kids' healthy energy. Remember, your life has an increased buzz to it; you are most likely working, cooking, cleaning, and trying to balance life with your family. Juicing is a great way for you to enjoy your daily antioxidants and to keep your energy up for your busy life. Amazingly, by just having a glass of homemade fresh fruit juice helps control sugar cravings. Another great attribute of consuming homemade raw vegetable juice is, you feel the energy rush or juice high without the drop of energy that you get after consuming a chocolate bar.

Pretty in Pink

I add Premier's pink salt to my juice, which helps with digestion, blood pressure and adrenals. Some people that suffer from digestive issues and vertigo have added pink salt and their symptoms disappeared. You can also buy either PINK Himalayan or sea salt from a health food store. Not only does consuming salt help keep us hydrated but studies show a deficiency in salt as a reason why some of us reach for the salted potato chips. Make sure you add pink salt to your juice or salt your food every day. Adults can use 1/4 to 1/2 tsp daily. Children over the age of two can enjoy 1/8 – 1/4 teaspoon of pink sea salt daily...not iodized white salt. Many kids use much more than that since high amounts of sodium hide in canned, frozen and processed foods, as well as the fast foods they consume every day. Please note that we are talking about homemade, mostly vegetable juice, NOT STORE BOUGHT commercial fruit or vegetable juice. Many of those juices contain sugar or corn syrup or are just concentrated fructose, excessively added sugar, the same sugar in that candy bar. Those vegetable juices contain very high levels of sodium, most using iodized salt to try and make it taste better. So don't be fooled...make it homemade. **Note: if you add pink salt, make sure you are not using high sodium commercial products like salted chips. Too much sodium can cause dehydration or other problems.**

Juicing helpful guidelines

- Vegetables should be as fresh as possible and organic
- Purchase at a local organic farm when possible

- Use as many leafy greens to enhance healing
- Purchase a juicer (low end – Jack LaLanne or Juiceman, or high end – Omega Vert 350)
- Use celery – nature's diuretic
- If you make extra juice, pour your juice into a wide-mouthed one-quart glass mason jars to store for the day (not with low end juicers that incorporate too much oxygen)
- Store your juice in a refrigerator
- Peel all vegetables that are not organic
- Clean all vegetables in limonene or polar mins (from Premier Research Labs)
- Raw juice has beneficial enzymes that give you the nutrients and energy to last throughout the day. I recommend raw juice to everyone, but especially if you are experiencing a time of stress or fatigue. Using a wide variety of vegetables and fruits will expose you to the widest range of minerals and vitamins
- Always use organic for produce listed on the dirty dozen and trim the exterior fruits and veggies that are on the clean 15 list (Chapter 3).

Juice & No Sugar Added Coconut Water Age 1 – 3

If you make a mostly fruit juice, thin it down with some unsweetened coconut water. If your juice contains many vegetables, you will not need to mix water with it.

- 1/2 cup coconut water
- 1/2 cup homemade fruit juice
- pinch pink sea salt

Juicy Fruit with Kale

- 1/2 cantaloupe
- 1 bunch of kale
- 1 orange
- 1 cucumber
- 1 green apples
- 1 lemon
- 1 cups pineapple
- 2 cups organic baby carrots

Joe Cross Incredible Juice Recipes

Find some great juice recipes at fatsickandnearlydead.com/about-the-film/learn-more/recipes. Watch his amazing transformation on his site.

Juicers

I use an Omega 350 Vertical Low Speed Masticating Juicer. The cost is around $380 – $425. The Omega's high-speed VRT350 juicer features the superior efficiency of a masticating style juicer in a vertical design. It is compact and productive. This juicer has a processing speed of 80 RPM. An oversized spout makes for easy serving. It weighs only 11 pounds, is stainless steel and easy to clean. The Omega has fine and coarse screens for pulp control; I use the fine screen since I prefer a small amount of pulp in my juice. The pulp from the juicer is dry, meaning it produces a larger yield of juice. This juicer can also handle wheatgrass, kale, spinach and collard greens. I make a gallon at a time which takes me an hour to make and clean up, and I can safely store my juice for three to four days. I consume at least a quart of juice a day (when not juice fasting). If you purchase a juicer you will need to cut up your celery in smaller pieces so it does not clog the juicer. In addition, when juicing softer foods like oranges, follow with harder veggies like carrots. If the machine stops and is clogged just reverse the on/off button and turn it back on to clear it out.

If you are at all concerned with the oxidation of your juices, or the rate at which they start to break down, it is important to buy a superior juicer over an average one. If you purchase a Jack LaLanne or Juiceman, you need to drink the juice immediately after making it. This is due to the oxidation or oxygen exposure. Although I believe a fresh, raw, organic juice is still a powerhouse of nutrition and enzymes, if you are suffering from a complicated health issue and are on a budget, buy the cheaper one and make and drink your juice daily. Oxidation occurs because of air (oxygen) exposure, which begins the process of breaking down the foods. A high quality juicer minimizes oxidation. Taking into consideration time requirements, your health realities and budget, you should be able to feel good about any decision you make concerning which method you choose to make your juice. Remember, the most important thing is drinking juice. Juice on!

When first serving fruit juice to young kids, mix with a 50% juice and 50% water or sugar free coconut water. As your kids get older, you can add less water and add more veggies. If you have a masticator juicer like an Omega Vert, you can store juice for up to 3 days.

Smoothies

If you cannot afford a juicer, then at least take advantage of a blender. A juicer takes out the fiber and pulp, which would digest into the colon as a normal process of digestion. However, juice does not digest; it metabolizes immediately, delivering antioxidants directly into the bloodstream. A smoothie made in a blender gives you the bulk needed for healthy digestion. Both are great ways to stay healthy.

An Apple a Day Smoothie

- 1 organic small sweet apple
- 1-2 organic kale leaves
- 1 peeled orange
- 1/4 peeled organic cucumber
- 1 cup unsweetened nut milk (cashew, almond, coconut) NOT SOY
- 1/8 tsp of pink sea salt

Bananas in Pajamas Smoothie

- 1/2 Banana
- 1 handful of organic spinach
- 3 baby organic carrots
- 1/2 cup of pineapple
- 1 cup nut milk
- 1/8 tsp pink sea salt

Almond Butter & Grape Jelly Belly

- 1 tbsp. of organic almond butter
- handful of organic spinach

- 1/2 peeled organic cucumber
- 1/2 cup of organic green grapes only
- 8 oz. nut milk
- 1/8 tsp pink sea salt

Over the Rainbow Smoothie

- 1 organic red apple
- 1 peeled orange
- 1-2 organic green kale leaves
- 1 yellow piece of pineapple
- 1 very small piece of red beet
- 1/8 tsp pink sea salt

Nutrients: Purchase from Premier Research Labs, Great to add into a smoothie for all kids but especially ones with health issues-7 months or older

- Add 1/4 cup Aloe Drink
- Add 1 tsp Greens Mix
- Add 1/2 tsp EFA Liquid
- Add 1/4 tsp coconut oil
- Add 1/2 tsp whey protein
- Add 1/2 tsp nutritional flakes
- Add 1/2 tsp Galactin
- Add 1/8 tsp Coral Legend
- Add 1 cap DHA
- Add 1/4 tsp Colostrum Powder

1 year ++++ Add the following to the above recipe.

- Week 1 add all of the above but now 1/4 tsp of Cod Liver Oil.
- Week 2 add all of the above plus 1/2 cup of Aloe Drink instead of 1/4.
- Week 3 add all of the above but now add 2 caps of DHA instead of 1.
- Week 4 add all of the above and a 1/2 tsp of Colostrum Powder instead of a 1/4 tsp.
- Gradually increase the dosage of the remaining products as needed for the child
- At about 1 1/2 years of age, 1/8 tsp Pink Salt daily

*Mom should also be on this (max dosage), through 18 months postpartum.

*This program is ideal for infants who have started on supplemental meals outside their breast feeding routine (no sooner than 7-9 months always check with your doctor).

Homemade nut milks

While almond milk is not exactly a superfood, there is nothing inherently unhealthy about it unless you choose varieties with added sweeteners or other additives. For the most part, it is more deceptive than anything, as you are paying a premium for mostly water and could get better nutrition from eating a handful of actual nuts. Still, it is a great milk substitute, tastes good and is fantastic as the base for a smoothie. If you want a "chunk full of nuts", making your own almond milk is far more economical, healthier, and has more nuts than buying the ready-made version.

You can increase the amount of almonds for added nutrition, leave out the sweeteners and other additives, and be left with an almond milk beverage that is good for your health at a fraction of the cost. It is simple to make, too.

Recipe for Homemade Almond Milk

- Soak about one cup of organic, raw almonds in cold water overnight (about 10-12 hours)
- Blend the almonds with about three cups of water (you can add more or less depending on how you like the consistency).
- Strain the frothy mixture through a cheesecloth, fine-mesh strainer or nut milk bag
- You can use walnuts instead of almonds. When using cashews, only soak for half an hour to make a quick and delicious milk.

Your almond milk will keep in the fridge for about three days (give it a stir before drinking). In addition, do not throw away the leftover pulp; it can be added to smoothies or even baked goods for added nutrition. One benefit to consuming almonds this way is that they will be soaked before you eat them. Soaking helps to get rid of the phytic acid and enzyme inhibitors, which can interfere with the function of your own digestive and metabolic enzymes.

Phytic acid, which is found in the coatings of nuts, is an "anti-nutrient" responsible for leaching vital nutrients from your body. Phytic acid also blocks the uptake of essential minerals such as calcium, magnesium, copper, iron, and zinc. Further, when nuts are soaked, the germination process begins, allowing the enzyme inhibitors to be deactivated and increasing the nutrition of the nut significantly, as well as making them much easier to digest. (Enzyme inhibitors in nuts [and seeds] help protect the nut as it grows, helping to decrease enzyme activity and prevent premature sprouting.)

It is a great idea to soak all raw nuts before eating them except raw cashews.

16

"CLOUDY WITH A CHANCE OF MEATBALLS" SERVING POISON ON YOUR PLATE

Antibiotics in Meat – You are Eating Sick Animals

From birth to slaughter, animals in production feedlots and all non-organic production sites, are given antibiotics constantly whether they are sick or not. This is done because these animals are raised in small cages, fed corn (making them sick) and some never see the light of day. Infections run rampant because of the overcrowding and dirty facilities. We already know that toxins are living in our organs, but many believe these hormones cause a host of problems for young girls reproductively. Every time you drink non-organic milk or eat non-organic meat, you are dosing yourself with a constant supply of antibiotics. What this means is that people are becoming more and more resistant to antibiotics, meaning you may need a stronger antibiotic when you do get sick.

"Where's the Beef"

Hopefully not on your plate unless it is organic!!! Limit the beef, chicken or pork to one time a week. *"Meet your maker"* and purchase your meat at your local butcher shop where they do not use hormones or antibiotics. There are so many toxins in today's mass produced meat such as: antibiotics, growth hormones, mad cow, E. coli, salmonella, pink slime, Bovine Viral Diarrhea, and Meat Glue.

When I was a child, all the farms produced grass-fed beef and the cows were not slaughtered until they were at least 4-5 years old. Cattle have evolved for millions of years to eat grass, but now they are corn fed. Corn makes them sick so they are given antibiotics. You may be eating a sick, corn fed cow. Greed is the reason. It is faster, but cows are slaughtered when they are less than 2 years old since many are so ill. Sick, cheap, fast food. Sound familiar? Start cleaning up your body, one organic hamburger or veggie burger at a time.

"Old MacDonald had a Farm, and on the Farm He Had a Pig" But Not Like This!

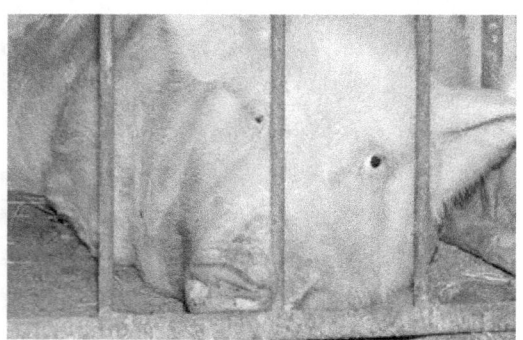

There have been a few changes with caged animals, where they are recommending cages be large enough for animals to turn around in. Please buy organic, knowing the animals you are eating were not abused.

Hormone Drugs - Serving Poison on Your Dinner Plate

It is a sin to see the cruel behavior used with our animals today. Animals are chemically injected with more and more toxins, forcing the size of the animal growth to *"plump up the volume."* It is becoming harder and harder to eat healthy. Here's how it works. Hormone drugs are manufactured as a pellet and are put under the skin of the animal's ear and discarded when they are slaughtered. It is hard to believe that in the U.S., all steroid hormone growth-promoting drugs are available as over-the-counter purchases. There are 6 FDA approved hormones for use in the beef industry, 3 synthetic and 3 natural. The 3 synthetic ones are melengestrol acetate, trenbolone acetate and zeranol and the 3 natural ones are estradiol, progesterone and testosterone. There are nearly 3,000 chemical additives are approved for use in food. Yikes!

Most traditionally raised beef calves go from 80 pounds to 1,200 pounds in a period of about 14 months. Wow that's fast! Today's cows are fed high quantities of corn and implanted with different drugs to fatten them up quickly.

Meat producers poison the animal from birth to death and you serve these chemicals to your family, your children's health is especially at risk. Some producers are now injecting the slaughtered meat with water, sodium phosphate and sodium to add tenderness and weight. There is no reason to buy NON-organic meat.

Measurable amounts of hormones in traditionally raised beef are transferred to humans, and some scientists believe that human consumption of estrogen from hormone-fed beef can result in cancer, premature puberty, and falling sperm counts.

FDA Wants Voluntary Decrease of Antibiotics Used,

Do You Think This Will Work?

The FDA revealed that sales of the two most commonly used antibiotics in livestock and poultry increased for the second consecutive year. Ranchers purchased 14.4 million pounds of penicillin and tetracycline in 2011, a 2.9 million pound increase from 2009. The U.S. Food and Drug Administration announced that they are "taking three steps to protect public health and promote the judicious use of medically important antibiotics in food-producing animals". The FDA issued a voluntary initiative to make some changes by issuing three documents that will help veterinarians, farmers and animal producers by limiting their antibiotic use to only address disease and health problems. If you voluntarily asked doctors to limit the use of drugs to patients do you think they would?

Organic Free Roaming - What's the difference

Organic free roaming outdoor animals have much stronger immune systems and seldom get sick. However, if one does get sick they are removed from the herd permanently if given antibiotics. Certified organic meats will not contain any antibiotics.

Animals raised for the purpose of providing certified organic meats are not allowed to eat any food which has been treated with synthetic fertilizers, pesticides, herbicides, sewage sludge or radiation. Their food sources cannot contain any preservatives, additives or GMO's. Organic grass fed cows are an excellent source of conjugated linoleic acid (CLA), and the meat is leaner and has a better fatty acid ratio. Research has found that raw dairy products and meat from grass fed cattle can have CLA levels at 30% to 50% higher than those of cattle fed a diet of primarily corn and grain. CLA has been found to reduce body fat, especially abdominal fat, combat Arteriosclerosis and help fight the onset of diabetes. CLA was found to improve insulin levels in about two-thirds of diabetic patients, and moderately reduced the blood glucose level and triglyceride levels. CLA reduces fat and preserves muscle tissue.

"We Don't Do Chickens Right"

The FDA has admitted some of chicken meat sold in the USA contains arsenic, a cancer-causing toxic chemical. The move follows a recent FDA study of 100 broiler chickens that detected inorganic arsenic, a known carcinogen, at higher levels in the livers of chickens treated with 3-Nitro, compared to untreated chickens. The U.S. Food and Drug Administration recently announced that Alpharma, a subsidiary of Pfizer Inc., will voluntarily suspend U.S. sales of the animal drug 3-Nitro (Roxarsone). American consumers who eat conventional chicken have been swallowing arsenic, a known cancer-causing chemical since 1940.

Gnaw on Some Raw

Cooked food is food that is cooked above 118 degrees for three minutes or longer. When cooked, the protein has become denatured and its sugar has become caramelized, and when the natural fibers have been broken down it is much harder to digest that food. When you eat cooked carbohydrates, proteins, and fats, you are eating numerous (carcinogenic) products caused by the cooking process. If you think of it, we are eating not just dead animals; we are really eating dead meat, lacking anything healthy for us.

Reasons Why You Should Not Eat a Lot of Cooked Food

- 80% of the vitamins and minerals are destroyed
- All of the enzymes are completely destroyed
- Pesticides become more toxic, oxygen is lost and free radicals are produced
- Digests in 40 – 100 hours
- Sleepiness after a meal
- Enormous increase of white blood cells (our warriors of defense, our
- immune system, which come out when we have infection or poisons)
- Quickly ferments and putrefies in the intestinal tract
- Causes allergy hyper-sensitivities
- Lose up to 97% of the water-soluble vitamins (Vitamins B and C)
- Lose up to 40% of the lipid soluble vitamins (Vitamins A, D, E and K)

"Gnaw on Some Raw"

- A *raw food* is a food that is not heated above 118 degrees (F).
- Contains lots of vitamins, minerals, enzymes, a live food
- Digests in 24 – 36 hours
- Raw food provides you with more strength, energy
- Stamina, memory and power of concentration
- Will have energy after a meal
- Usually sleep better
- No increase in white blood cells, which rush in after eating
- Raw foods do not spoil quickly
- Elimination of body odor and halitosis

"I Tawt I Taw a Puddy Tat"

Well, if you are not convinced let's look at one of my favorite studies, the Pottinger study of **900 cats over a ten year period**. This study is broken down into 2 groups:

Group #1 - fed an all raw diet; raw milk, raw meat and cod liver oil, lived in all four generations and only 5% developed degenerative/ human diseases.

Group #2 - fed cooked meat, raw milk and cod liver oil. The cooked group was sick later in life in the first generation, many born with disease and blind, and **all cats died out in the fourth generation.**

So why am I telling you about a cat study and a raw diet? If the cats ate a healthy raw diet, they produced healthy offspring, but for those that had unhealthy diet of cooked food, they got sicker with each generation, eventually dying out. Sooooo, if you are unhealthy maybe your chances of producing a healthy baby are not as probable. As far as the raw component, I am simply stating facts; the cats lived healthy lives on all raw. It just makes sense. If you need to improve your health, are you going to reach for a hamburger or a salad?

17

"FINDING NEMO" FISH TAILS AND TALES

Fish farming is the raising of fish commercially in tanks or enclosures in small spaces. There are also fish hatcheries where young fish are raised in a tank and then released into the wild to be recaptured later. The most popular farm raised fish include, salmon, carp, tilapia and catfish. Farm raised fish and seafood equals a cesspool of toxic and dangerous chemicals you ingest through the food. Most supermarket fish are farm-raised, meaning that they use higher concentrations of antibiotics. Research has shown that farm raised fish also have a 20% lower protein content. Farm raised are given antibiotics to treat disease for over-crowded pool conditions. It seems over-crowded habitats for farm animals produce the same results. There has been extensive commercialization and increased consumption of aquaculture seafood products worldwide.

The FDA states, "aqua-cultured seafood has become the fastest growing sector of the world food economy, accounting for approximately half of all seafood production worldwide. Approximately 80% of the seafood consumed in the U.S. is imported from approximately 62 countries. Over 40% of that seafood comes from aquaculture operations. As the aquaculture industry continues to grow and compete with wild-caught seafood products, concerns regarding the use of unapproved animal drugs and unsafe chemicals and the misuse of animal drugs in aquaculture operations have increased substantially". "China is the largest producer of aqua-cultured seafood in the world, accounting for 70% of the total production and 55% of the total value of aqua-cultured seafood exported around the world. The use of unapproved antibiotics or chemicals in aquaculture raises significant public health concerns."

The FDA quoted on their website that studies show "the seafood from China has a high percentage of contaminants and that in 2008 they were going to put a broader import control on all farm raised fish, shrimp, carp and eel from China". Do not wait, check the labels, and do not check out with farm raised fish, only wild caught.

Fish Recommendations

Even though the list below contains the mercury levels of fish and seafood, there are other considerations on how fish are caught and killed, if they are farm raised or wild caught, or what other types of feed these sea creatures ingest. The following are recommendations from Dr. Marshall from Premier Research Labs.

Dr. Marshall's Most Recommended (Wild Caught)

1. Dover Sole
2. Halibut
3. Swai
4. Whitefish
5. Sardines
6. Anchovies
7. Cordina
8. Mackerel
9. Haddock
10. Red Snapper

Dr. Marshall's Less Desirable -Don't Eat or Eat Less Often

Salmon
Flounder
Sea Bass
Shrimp
Tilapia
Trout
Catfish
Mahi Mahi
Cod
Herring
Shark
Tuna
Albacore
Crab
Lobster
Scallops

The following is a list of fish and seafood and their mercury content from least to most mercury. The categories on the list were determined according to the following mercury levels in the flesh of tested fish.

- Least mercury: Less than 0.09 parts per million
- Moderate mercury: From 0.09 to 0.29 parts per million
- High mercury: From 0.3 to 0.49 parts per million
- Highest mercury: More than .5 parts per million

Least Mercury

Anchovies
Butterfish
Catfish
Clam
Crab (Domestic)
Crawfish/Crayfish
Croaker (Atlantic)
Flounder
Haddock (Atlantic)
Hake
Herring
Mackerel (N. Atlantic)
Mullet
Oyster
Perch (Ocean)
Plaice
Pollock
Salmon (Fresh)
Sardine
Scallop
Shad (American)
Shrimp
Sole (Pacific)
Squid (Calamari)
Tilapia
Trout (Freshwater)
Whitefish
Whiting

Moderate Mercury - Eat six servings or less per month:

Bass (Striped, Black)
Carp
Cod (Alaskan)
Croaker (White Pacific)
Halibut (Atlantic)
Halibut (Pacific)
Jacksmelt
(Silverside)
Lobster
Mahi Mahi
Monkfish
Perch (Freshwater)
Sablefish
Skate
Snapper
Tuna (canned chunk light)
Tuna (Skipjack)
Weakfish (Sea Trout)

High Mercury - Eat three servings or less per month:

Bluefish
Grouper
Mackerel (Spanish, Gulf)
Sea Bass (Chilean)
Tuna (Canned Albacore)
Tuna (Yellowfin)

Highest Mercury - Avoid eating:

Mackerel (King)
Marlin
Orange Roughy
Shark
Swordfish
Tilefish
Tuna (Bigeye, Ahi)

Sources for NRDC's guide: The data for this guide to mercury in fish comes from two federal agencies: The Food and Drug Administration, which tests fish for mercury, and the Environmental Protection Agency, which determines mercury levels that it considers safe for women of childbearing age.

18

"*RUB A DUB DUB*" CLEANING PRODUCTS

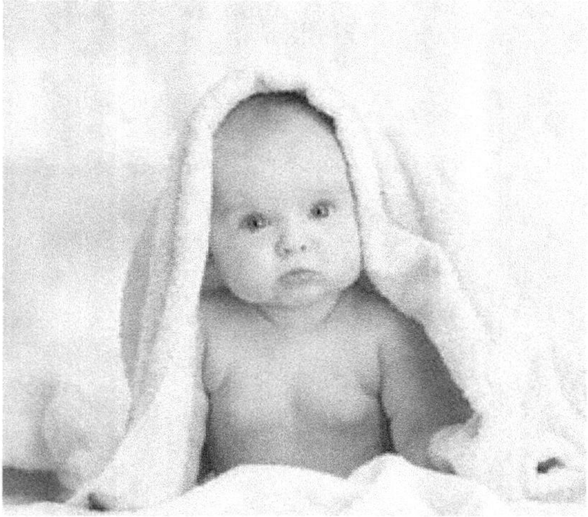

Your newborn is very sensitive as their organs are still developing when they are first born. Imagine when you first bring your baby home from the hospital. You think you have done an incredible job of cleaning your home, especially your baby's room. You bleach the sheets, use fabric sheets in the dryer with formaldehyde, use chemical cleaners to clean the room, window cleaners and air fresheners. You think you are cleaning up when really you are providing a toxic environment for your newborn. As they grow, they crawl on the floor and are constantly putting their hands in their mouth. When they go outside to play at home, daycares or schools, they are running, rolling and placing their hands on the newly chemically treated lawns. When they go to school, they are sitting at desks, lunch tables and using rest rooms that have been cleaned with harmful chemicals, especially bleach.

Take a trash bag and throw out the toxic cleaners under your kitchen sink, around the washer and dryer, in your garage and basement, your linen closet. Go Green and buy cleaners without the toxins or use vinegar and water! They work as well as the toxic chemicals and are much healthier for your family.

There are so many toxins that we breathe, apply, eat and drink every day. When you consider how many we are exposed to collectively (daily, weekly, yearly), you will see that as we age we have accumulated a lifetime of toxins. In today's world, it is impossible to avoid all toxins, but it is imperative that we learn healthy alternatives to keep our toxins at bay.

EPA states 87,000 different chemicals are now in use in homes, industry and agriculture.

No Labeling of Contents for Cleaning Products Is Required By Law

Rebecca Sutton, PhD, a senior scientist at the Environmental Working Group (EWG), explains, "In terms of household cleaners, neither ingredients nor products must meet any sort of safety standard, nor is any testing data or notification required before bringing a product to market."

"The average household contains about 62 toxic chemicals, say environmental experts. We are exposed to them routinely — from the phthalates in synthetic fragrances to the noxious fumes in oven cleaners. Ingredients in common household products have been linked to asthma, cancer, reproductive disorders, hormone disruption and neurotoxicity."

We are in the dark - What's Missing? - The Ingredients!

EWG researched more than 2,000 common cleaning products. Manufacturers can use nearly any substance they want, hiding information about the toxic ingredients from consumers. Cleaning products, unlike foods, beverages, cosmetics and other personal care products are not required by federal law to carry a list of ingredients. The manufacturers have no restrictions to avoid risky chemicals even if they can trigger asthma attacks or are linked to disease.

Dangerous Products We Use Everyday

Mercury

Metallic mercury is a shiny, odorless liquid. When heated it produces an odorless poisonous gas. Mercury spills can occur in hospitals and science classrooms. Sadly, mercury amalgams are still being put into children's teeth, which is a constant dose of mercury. The vapors from mercury can be inhaled and cause respiratory problems, especially asthma.

Found in:

- Thermometers
- Barometers
- Batteries
- Mercury amalgam fillings
- Fish

The Agency for Toxic Substances and Disease Registry (ATSDR) from the CDC states, acute exposure to vapors from metallic mercury can result in the following:

Dangers: "Respiratory distress, increased blood pressure, and gastrointestinal effects (nausea, vomiting, and diarrhea). Long term effects include brain and nervous system issues, causing irritability, tremors, and/or memory problems.

Dangers: "to very young children include damage to the brain, kidneys, and developing fetus".

Formaldehyde

There is usually more formaldehyde present indoors than outdoors. Formaldehyde is released to the air from many home products and you may breathe in formaldehyde while using these products. You may also be affected by touching or absorption into the pours of our skin.

Found In:

- Latex paint, fingernail hardener, and fingernail polish
- Plywood, particle board, furniture and cabinets
- Unvented gas or kerosene heaters - indoors
- Smoke from a cigar, cigarette, or pipe - indoors
- New carpet, decorative laminate flooring
- Lacquers, insulations, adhesives
- Some permanent press fabrics
- Grocery bags and paper towels
- Household cleaners, carpet cleaners, disinfectants
- Cosmetics, medicines and vaccines
- Fabric softeners, kids glue, and antiseptics

Dangers: It has been shown to cause cancer of the upper airways, leukemia, and respiratory illness.

Phthalates

Phthalates are in many fragranced household products such as air fresheners, dish soap, even toilet paper. If you see the word "fragrance" on a label, there is a good chance phthalates are present. According to the CDC, when phthalates are absorbed through the skin they go straight to organs since the skin has no protection from these toxins.

Found In

- Food and liquid containers
- Baby formula & baby food

- Pesticides
- Cosmetics, personal care products, perfumes
- Infant care products
- Medications
- Medical devices
- Shower curtains, flooring, wall paper, mini blinds
- Diaper mats, rain gear, school supplies
- Car interiors, inflatable mattresses
- Dangerous shower curtains with (BPA)

Dangers: These are endocrine disruptors and can be dangerous to a developing child. It can damage the liver, kidneys, lungs, and reproductive system, and in the development of the testes which can cause a reduction in the sperm count.

Healthier Choices: When you have something plastic, look at the little triangle on the bottom of the container. Avoiding plastic containers marked with a 1,3,6 or 7, and instead choose those marked with a 2, 4, or 5 which will reduce the likelihood of exposure to BPA and phthalates. Avoid most of these products, including shower curtains.

Environmental Protection Agency (EPA) found "off-gassing toxins: phthalates, toluene, ethylbenzene, phenol, methyl isobutyl ketone, xylene, acetophenone and cumene from shower curtains". From one of the curtains, there were up to 108 VOC's (volatile organic compounds) leached into the air that remained airborne for almost one month. The inhalation of these toxins (yup, it's in that **new shower curtain** smell) over time, can cause anything from headaches and nausea to liver, central nervous system, respiratory and reproductive problems.

There are PEVA (polyethylene vinyl acetate) and EVA (ethylene vinyl acetate) which are made from petrochemicals (petroleum and natural gas) which are still a fossil fuel pollutant, but they contain less VOC's than PVC's. PEVA/EVA choices are chlorine-free which have been shown to considerably reduce harmful off gassing. So buy PVC, PEVA/EVA Free, hemp, linen, and organic cotton.

Triclosan

Triclosan is an aggressive antibacterial agent that can promote the growth of drug-resistant bacteria.

Found In:

- Most liquid dishwashing detergents
- Hand soaps labeled "antibacterial."
- Ammonium compounds
- Fabric softener liquids and sheets
- Household cleaners labeled "antibacterial"

Dangers: The EPA is currently investigating whether Triclosan may also disrupt endocrine (hormonal) function. It is a probable carcinogen, suspected as a culprit for respiratory disorders.

Healthier Choice:

a. Use white vinegar in the rinse cycle to help prevent static cling.
b. Alternatives to chemical disinfectants abound, including antibacterial, antifungal tea-tree oil. Mix a few drops of tea-tree oil and a tablespoon of vinegar with water in a spray bottle for a safe, germ killing, all-purpose cleaner. Add a couple of drops of lavender essential oil for scent.

Butoxyethanol

2-butoxyethanol is the key ingredient found in many window cleaners, giving them their characteristic sweet smell. This powerful solvent causes dangers if inhaled.

Found In:

- Window, kitchen and multipurpose cleaners
- Ammonia
- Polishing agents for bathroom fixtures and sinks
- Jewelry cleaner

Dangers: Causes sore throats when inhaled, at high levels glycol ethers can also contribute to narcosis, pulmonary edema, and severe liver and kidney damage.

Healthier Choice: Clean mirrors and windows with newspaper and diluted vinegar. Make your own formulas with baking soda, vinegar and essential oils. Purchase Norwex clothes which clean with water only. These are my personal favorites. They are the best window and mirror cleaners, streak free.

Ammonia

Ammonia is a powerful irritant that when inhaled, especially with asthma patients, elderly, COPD and other lung issues and breathing problems. Bacteria, decaying plants and animals, and animal waste produce it naturally.

Found In:

- Glass and window cleaner
- Toilet bowl cleaner
- Oven cleaner
- Drain cleaner
- Multi-purpose cleaner

Dangers: Can cause chronic bronchitis and Asthma

NEVER MIX Ammonia and Bleach - can create a poisonous gas

Heathier Choice: Toothpaste as a jewelry cleaner, vinegar and water for glass, and Norwex for clothes

Chlorine

Chlorine can be inhaled through cleaning products, drank through water, and absorbed through your skin when you shower. It can be found in:

- Scouring powders
- Toilet bowl cleaners
- Mildew removers
- Laundry whiteners
- Household tap water

Dangers: Can cause chronic and acute respiratory problems and is a thyroid disrupter

Healthier Choice: Use Bon Ami or baking soda. Toilet bowls can be cleaned with vinegar. Vinegar or borax powder both work well for whitening clothes. It is essential to install filters under your sink and in all bathroom shower faucets.

Sodium Hydroxide

Sodium hydroxide is very dangerous. It can cause severe burning if it touches your skin or gets in your eyes. Inhalation can cause a source throat and respiratory problems especially for people with asthma.

Found In:

- Oven cleaners
- Drain openers

Healthier Choice: Combine 1-cup baking soda with a little vinegar and make into a paste to clean your oven. Combine 1-cup vinegar and 1-cup baking soda and pour down clogged drain. Wait 30 minutes and run hot water for at least 2 minutes to clear.

Toxic/Poison

Stay away from these items. They poison or damage your body: solvents, batteries, wood stains and polyurethane, antifreeze, radiator coolants, pesticides, fertilizers, preservatives, and compact fluorescent light bulbs.

Corrosive

These items eat away at surfaces, including your skin. Corrosive materials include: bleach, ammonia, rust removers, drain cleaners, laundry stain removers, glue removers, oven cleaners, and automotive lead-acid batteries.

Flammable

Anything that is flammable will burn easily with a minimal spark or heat. They include fuel oil, gasoline, motor oil, kerosene, camping fuel, paint thinners, lighter fluids, oil-based paints, insect repellent, aerosol containers, turpentine, and gasoline/oil mixtures, and contact cement.

Fragrance – Cleaners, Perfumes, Musk's

The International Fragrance Association, an industry trade group, acknowledges that the scents added to cleaners and other consumer goods may contain any number of more than 3,000 different chemical ingredients (IFRA 2010). Many have harmful ingredients such as linalool, eugenol, phthalates and synthetic musk's.

Healthier Choice: When possible, choose fragrance-free or all-natural organic products. Stop using aerosol products and plug-in air fresheners and instead use essential oils and diffusers for a constant spray of scent. Bring the outside in by opening windows and adding plants to help purify the air.

Perchloroethylene or PERC

Perc is a neurotoxin, according to the chief scientist of environmental protection for the New York Attorney General's office. EPA classifies perc as a "possible carcinogen".

Found in:

- Dry-cleaning solutions
- Spot removers
- Carpet and upholstery cleaners

Health Risks: Dizziness, loss of coordination

Healthier Choice: Avoid Dry Cleaning; use a wet cleaner instead. If you have to, dry clean, make sure to air them out before bringing them into your home.

Remove from Your Home - Candles

Simply put, many scented candles are toxic. Almost half of all scented candles on the market today contain lead wiring in their wicks, which is released into the air upon burning, leading to hormone disruption, behavioral disorders, and various other health problems. Be wary of candles made with paraffin wax, which generates two highly toxic compounds when burned: benzene and toluene, both of which are known carcinogens. Many scented candles contain artificial fragrances and dyes, which end up in your lungs when you burn them.

Healthy Choice: Buy a diffuser and use essential oils.

The Environmental Working Group (EWG) is one of the best resources to explore toxic substances and healthy alternatives to help you reduce your toxic load. The following is a list of alternatives to your favorite household products. I only posted the items that scored an A by the EWG. Go to their site and you can type in any brand name of cleaners to cosmetics to see how the products you are using rate.

Air Fresheners

- Arm & Hammer Fridge & Freezer Baking Soda
- Aussan Natural room odor eliminator
- Aura Cacia Aromatherapy Mist, Eucalyptus Harvest
- Aura Cacia Precious Essentials Aromatherapy Spritz, Purifying Sandalwood
- Aussan Natural nursery odor eliminator
- Arm & Hammer Fridge Fresh Refrigerator Air Filter
- Earth Friendly Products Uni-Fresh Air Freshener, Vanilla Scent

- Aura Cacia Aromatherapy Mist, Peppermint Harvest, Tangerine Grapefruit, Ginger Mint

All Purpose Cleaners

- Bon Ami Powder Cleanser
- Dr. Bronner's Sal Suds Liquid Cleaner
- Sun & Earth All Purpose Cleaner, Light Citrus
- Ecover Cream Scrub
- Dr. Bronner's Pure-Castile Soap, Peppermint
- Arm & Hammer Baking Soda
- Dr. Bronner's 18-in-1 Hemp Pure-Castile Soap Baby Mild
- Biokleen All Purpose Cleaner Concentrate
- Earth Friendly Products Orange Plus All Purpose Everyday Cleaner
- Ballard Organics All-Purpose Concentrated Liquid Soap, Jasmine / Bergamot
- Aussan Natural all-purpose cleaner
- Attitude All Purpose Eco Cleaner
- Aussan Natural nursery all-purpose cleaner
- Heinz Vinegar Distilled White Vinegar
- Arm & Hammer Super Washing Soda Detergent Booster & Household Cleaner
- Whole Foods Market all-purpose cleaner, citrus
- Whole Foods Market all-purpose concentrated cleaner, pine
- Imus GTC Greening the Cleaning All Purpose Cleaner, Citrus Sage
- Green Shield Organic Biodegradable Surface Wipes, Fresh
- Green Shield Organic All-Purpose Cleaner Degreaser, Fresh
- Disinfectant Scoring an A (only one)
- Seventh Generation Disinfecting Multi-Surface Cleaner, Lemongrass Citrus

Dusting Products Scored a C (no A's or B's)

- Pledge Multi Surface Duster, Fragrance Free

General Purpose

- Bon Ami Powder Cleanser
- Dr. Bronner's Sal Suds Liquid Cleaner
- Sun & Earth All Purpose Cleaner, Light Citrus
- Ecover Cream Scrub
- Dr. Bronner's Pure-Castile Soap, Peppermint
- Arm & Hammer Baking Soda
- Dr. Bronner's 18-in-1 Hemp Pure-Castile Soap Baby Mild
- Biokleen All Purpose Cleaner Concentrate
- Earth Friendly Products Orange Plus All Purpose Everyday Cleaner
- Ballard Organics All-Purpose Concentrated Liquid Soap, Jasmine / Bergamot

Glass Cleaners

- Citra-Solv Citra Clear Window & Glass Cleaner
- Simple Green Naturals Glass & Surface Care, Rosemary Mint
- Sun & Earth Glass Cleaner, Light Citrus
- Attitude Window & Mirror Eco Cleaner
- Whole Foods Market glass cleaner, unscented
- Green Shield Organic Glass Cleaner, Fresh
- Ology Glass Cleaner
- AspenClean Glass Cleaner
- Murchison-Hume Premium Glass Polish, Fragrance Free

Graffiti/Stain Remover No A,B,C,D only F's

- none

Mold and Mildew Remover Products

- Concrobium Mold Control
- Attitude Bathroom Mold & Mildew Cleaner

Bathroom Cleaners

- Green Shield Organic Bathroom Cleaner, Fresh
- BuggyLOVE Organic Multi-Surface Bathroom Cleaner, Clementine Scent
- AspenClean Bathroom Cleaner
- Seventh Generation Natural Tub & Tile Cleaner, Emerald Cypress & Fir
- Seventh Generation Natural Toilet Bowl Cleaner, Emerald Cypress & Fir
- Earth Friendly Products Toilet Cleaner, Natural Cedar Scent
- Green Shield Organic Toilet Bowl Cleaner
- MamaSuds Toilet Bombs
- Earth Friendly Products Shower Cleaner
- CLR Calcium, Lime, Rust Cleaner

Dishwashing Products

- Attitude Little Ones Baby Bottle & Dishwashing Liquid, Fragrance Free
- Earth Friendly Products Wave Auto Dishwasher Gel, Organic Lavender
- Browse Seventh Generation Automatic Dishwasher Powder, Free & Clear
- Seventh Generation Automatic Dishwasher Detergent Concentrated Pacs, Free & Clear
- Biokleen Automatic Dish Powder, Citrus Essence
- Earth Friendly Products Wave Auto Dishwasher Gel, Free & Clear
- Biokleen Automatic Dish Gel
- Sun & Earth Dishwashing Liquid Extra Concentrated, Light Citrus
- Green Shield Organic Squeeze Automatic Dishwasher Liquid Detergent, Lemongrass
- The Honest Co. honest auto dishwasher gel, free & clear

Floor Care Cleaners

- Earth Friendly Products Concentrated Carpet Shampoo with Bergamot and Sage
- Simple Green Naturals Carpet Care
- Martha Stewart Clean Carpet Stain Remover
- Fit Organic Laundry & Carpet Stain Remover
- Simple Green Naturals Floor Care
- Aussan Natural floor cleaner concentrate
- Babyganics Floor Cleaner Concentrate, Fragrance Free
- Martha Stewart Clean Wood Floor Cleaner
- Truce Wood Cleaner, Citrus
- Truce Wood Cleaner Concentrate Refills, Citrus

Furniture Cleaners

- BuggyLOVE Organic No-Wash Stain Remover, Tangerine Scent
- BuggyLOVE Organic Stroller & Carseat Fabric Cleaner, Clementine Scent
- Earth Friendly Products Everyday Stain & Odor Remover
- Aussan Natural nursery odor eliminator
- Eco-Me Carpet Freshener, Matt
- Attitude Little Ones Fabric Refresher, Fragrance Free
- LA's Totally Awesome Power Oxygen Base Cleaner
- Babyganics Stain Eraser, Fragrance Free
- Martha Stewart Clean Wood Floor Cleaner
- Truce Wood Cleaner, Citrus

Kitchen Cleaners

- BuggyLOVE Organic Multi-Surface Kitchen Cleaner, Tangerine Scent
- AspenClean Kitchen Cleaner
- Green Shield Organic All-Purpose Cleaner Degreaser, Fresh
- Whole Foods Market green MISSION Organic All-Purpose Spray Cleaner & Degreaser, Lemon Zest
- Fit Organic Cleaner and Degreaser
- Earth Friendly Products OXO Brite Non-Chlorine Bleach
- Ecover Non-Chlorine Bleach Powder
- Ecover Non-Chlorine Bleach Liquid
- Seventh Generation Chlorine Free Bleach, Free & Clear
- Biokleen Oxygen Bleach Plus
- Nature Clean Oxygen Bleach
- Arm & Hammer Super Washing Soda Detergent Booster & Household Cleaner
- OxiClean Laundry Baby Stain Soaker
- GrabGreen Bleach Alternative Pods, Fragrance Free
- Sun & Earth on the Spot! Instant Stain Remover

Baby and Pet Products that Scored A

- BuggyLOVE Organic Stroller Frame & Accessory Cleaner, Sweet Orange Scent
- Aussan Natural cat odor eliminator
- Aussan Natural dog odor eliminator
- Attitude Little Ones Toy & Surface Cleaner, Fragrance Free
- Babyganics All Purpose Surface Wipes, Fragrance Free
- Dr. Bronner's Pure-Castile Soap, Baby Unscented
- Fit Organic Baby Laundry Detergent
- Fit Organic Baby Laundry Stain Remover

"The EPA has classified some forms of mercury (both organic and inorganic) as "possible human Carcinogens". About 1 in 10 children in the United States has asthma. Asthmagens are substances that can cause asthma in people who have never had asthma before. Specific asthmagens include ingredients found in many cleaning and disinfecting products. These products include acid cleansers, disinfectants, carpet cleaners, floor strippers, ammonia, and graffiti removers. Cleaning and disinfecting product ingredients that are asthmagens include bleach, quaternaryammonium compounds, ethanolamines, ammonia, acids, etc."

19

"SPONGEBOB SQUAREPANTS" TOXIC DIAPERS

In our fast-paced society, most Mommies go back to work after 6 weeks to 3 months. That means packing up a bag to take to the sitter/day care. We throw in some disposable diapers, preferred pumped breast milk, disposable wipes, and baby lotion. Your baby will be using them 24/7 for the next few years. Most disposable diapers contain harmful chemicals, dyes, bleaching and fragrances that will be absorbed through breathing and through the vaginal area for girls.

Sodium Polyacrylate

Sodium polyacrylate is a super absorbent chemical added to diapers in a granular powder that is used in the fillers of many disposable diapers. It turns into a gel when it mixes with urine and can absorb 300 times its weight in water. This chemical was removed from tampons due to "toxic shock syndrome" but has been used in diapers for the last 20 years.

Dangers: It is a skin irritant, a drying agent; it leaches oil and moisture from baby's skin. Exposure to respirable dust may cause respiratory tract and lung irritation and may aggravate existing respiratory conditions.

Toxins from Bleaching (Dioxins)

The chlorine bleach process leaves behind toxins in the fibers called "dioxins." Dioxins are extremely toxic and can cause problems in the endocrine systems (hormones), infertility later in life and are cancer causing Dioxins and sodium Polyacrylate, two of the chemicals found in disposable diapers.

Dioxins and Sodium Polyacrylate, two of the chemicals found in disposable diapers, have been linked to have caused the following:

Danger toxic responses: induce a wide spectrum of toxic responses in experimental animals: cancer, reproductive & infertility problems, asthma & respiratory distress, developmental (developmental delays and changes in the development of the fetus hormonal problems), developmental & cognitive problems, suppressed immune system, diabetes, endometriosis, allergic reactions, chemical burns.

Tributyl-tin (TBT)

Many disposable diapers contain a chemical called tributyl-tin (TBT). According to the EPA, this toxic pollutant is **extremely harmful to aquatic (water) life** and causes **endocrine (hormonal) disruptions** in aquatic organisms. It is linked to obesity in humans (triggers genes that cause the growth of fat cells).

Volatile Organic Compounds (VOCs)

Disposable diapers frequently contain chemicals called volatile organic compounds (VOCs). These include chemicals such as ethylbenzene (Styrene), toluene, and xylene. According to the EPA, VOCs can cause eye, nose and throat irritation, **headaches, damage to the liver, kidneys and central nervous system**. Some VOCs are even suspected of causing **cancer** in humans (EPA.gov).

Dyes, Fragrances, Plastics and Petroleum's

Fragrances: contain phthalates, the class of chemicals known to disrupt the endocrine system.

Petroleum: Petrolatum is a soft paraffin or wax mixture sold and acknowledged by the U.S. Food and Drug Administration as an approved over-the-counter skin protectant. Side effects include finding the petroleum byproduct in breast tumors, suffocation of the skin, and premature aging and aggravated acne.

Dyes and plastics have both been discussed in the chapter for ADHD/ADD.

Conventional, Disposable Diapers

Many new mommies have already had a baby showers and the babies' rooms are already stacked with the conventional diapers like Pampers and Huggies. Remember companies do not need to show the ingredients on diapers. Huggies has a pure and natural organic cotton on the outside of the diaper but still uses chlorine.

This is what we do not want: sodium polyacrylate or SAP, volatile organic compounds or VOCs (including toluene, ethylbenzene, xylene, and dipentene), dioxins, polyurethane, adhesives, lotions, inks, fragrances, and pesticide residue.

"Natural" Disposables

Following is a list of diaper companies using fewer chemicals than the conventional ones. These are better options, limiting the amount of chemicals next to your baby's delicate skin:

Seventh Generation, Earth's Best, Nurtured by Nature - Made primarily with natural ingredients (as opposed to synthetic), use minimal processing, and are free of chlorine, latex, fragrance, dyes, and lotions.

Nature Babycare - Made from natural materials, free of chlorine, latex, fragrance, dyes, and lotions. They use absorbent pulp from sustainably harvested forests, GMO-free corn and no plastic.

Honest Company: These are free of chlorine, latex, lotions, fragrance phthalates, optical brighteners, PVC, heavy metals, organotins (MBT, DBT, TBT), and harsh petrochemical additives. The chlorine-free pulp is sustainably harvested and the plant-based inner and outer layers reduce added petrochemicals. The inner core is made from BIO-based wheat/corn, with reduced SAP.

Attitude: Chlorine free, fragrance free, made from vegetable based materials, biodegradable inner shell and padding, and CO2 neutral.

Bamboo Nature: These are certified free of "all" dangerous chemicals, including chlorine, phthalates, organotin, heavy metals, formaldehyde, colophonium, AZO-pigments, and PVC. Bamboo Nature diapers are also free of all known allergens and substances classified as skin irritants, sensitizing, carcinogenic, or mutagenic. To boot these diapers are 75% biodegradable and 99% compostable, and all wood pulp is derived from sustainable tree farms.

Broody Chick: These are all chlorine free, SAP (Sodium Polyacrylate) free, fragrance free, G.E. (genetically free) free, biodegradable and compostable.

Hybrid Diapers

Hybrid diapers are a little more flexible, eco-friendly and have nontoxic alternative to disposable diapers. Hybrids include brands like gDiapers, GroVia, and Flip. They offer the option of an outer shell that can be worn multiple times before washing with either a biodegradable disposable insert or a washable cloth insert. Hybrids combine disposables with reusable cloth diapers covers.

Cloth Diapers- The Best Choice

The cloth diaper market is thriving, includes many types of materials and offer parent peace of mind with chemical free alternatives. There are flats, prefolds, contours, fitted, pockets, and all-in-ones to choose from. These come in many variations of materials including:

White Cotton – These are bleached and leave toxins in the fibers, Dioxins. The unhealthiest choice.

Organic cotton - Organic Cotton (unbleached and dye-free) Cloth Diapers. Unbleached with no chemicals. Free of sodium polyacrylate/super absorbent polymer. Buy the ones that use absorbent cotton layers, an absorbent liner and a breathable diaper cover.

Bamboo (unbleached and dye-free) Cloth Diapers – Bamboo is less bulky and softer and more absorbent than cotton. Bamboo is broken down into pulp, chemically processed and aged, then forced out as a rayon fiber. It is a woody plant that grows easily without pesticides and fungicides. Bamboo is softer than hemp but not as absorbent as hemp.

Hemp (unbleached and dye-free) Cloth Diapers. It is a woody plant that grows easily without pesticides and fungicides. The hemp fibers spun into yarn are the natural fibers from the plant. Hemp is mechanically processed, aided by natural enzymes and chemicals. This long process involves many chemicals. Hemp is not as soft as bamboo and cotton but more absorbent.

There is also chlorine-free paper pulp as an absorbent layer to add to diapers that are fragrance-free and hypoallergenic

Natural Diaper Resources

Babyworks -- Organic and natural fiber cloth diapers, (800)422-2910.

California Babestuff -- Cloth diapers and other accessories, (804)988-6888.

Diaperaps, Ltd. -- Cloth diapers and diapering accessories, (800)477-3424.

Ecobaby Organics, Inc. -- Cloth diapers and organic baby clothing and bedding, (619)562-9606.

Katie's Kisses -- Organic cotton diapers and hemp diapers, (888)881-0404.

Mama's Earth -- Organic cotton diapers, bedding and clothing, (800)620-7388.

Under the Nile -- Organic Egyptian cotton diapers and more, (800)883-4402.

What's Hempenin' Baby -- Hemp cloth diapers and more, (740)694-4442.
Xanomi -- Organic cotton diapers and more, (800)442-9046.

Cloth Diapering Tips

Go Leak-Free: Cloth diapers now come in different sizes, with snap and Velcro closures and fitted leg openings, and can be tucked inside a cloth and vinyl "diaper cover" for extra leak protection.

Purchase thin, unbleached, 100 percent biodegradable paper liners so you can just flush down the toilet. Make your life safer and easier and your baby healthier.

For overnight protection, many companies sell organic cotton "diaper doublers," a thick piece of cloth you can tuck inside a cloth diaper for extra absorbency.

Natural Fiber Cloth Diapers — Diapers containing hemp, bamboo, or natural cotton need to be washed and dried around 3 to 6 times before using. This rinses out the natural oils contained in the fibers.

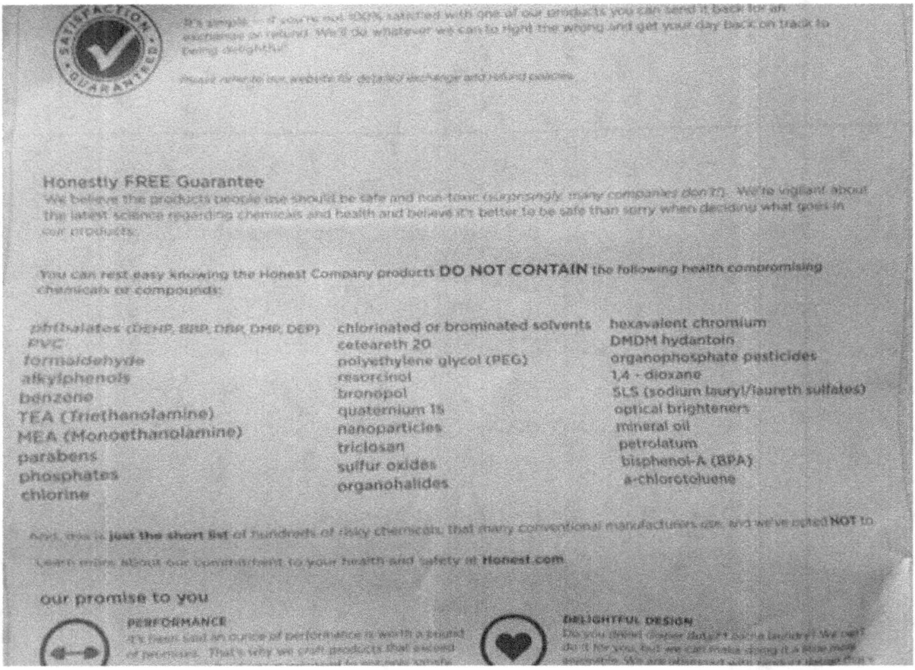

When to Wash

It is best to wash diapers every 2 days. If you wait any longer, urine-soaked diapers will lock in ammonia and microorganisms have greater opportunity to grow creating persistent odor issues and potential for diaper rash.

Where do I put the diaper?

Wet Bags or pail liners are the most popular storage devices. Wet bags come in many different sizes and hanging options. Pail liners are the perfect size to use like a trash bag in a trashcan (or similar sized container.) It can even be used without a pail. You can use a hamper with holes in it. Wet diapers should be stored in a dry well ventilated room with the best airflow away from pets and kids. Do not soak your diapers as it can cause a cesspool of bacteria. It is a good idea to rinse diapers out before putting them in a diaper pail. If you use a wet bag or a pail liner you should be washing it with every diaper wash load. If you use a laundry basket, you should wipe it clean every wash as well.

How to Wash Cloth Diapers

Mainly wash on Hot (Pre-wash temp is personal preference)

Use 1x the recommended amount in your pre-rinse/pre-wash

Use 1.5-2x the recommended amount in the main wash

The following is Real Diaper Association's best practice Cloth Diaper Laundry Guide that is based upon the idea that before drying, all detergent residues should be thoroughly rinsed away. That is, in the final rinse, there should be no lingering suds.

Rinse warm

Wash hot with detergent (a longer cycle)

Rinse warm twice

Machine Dry on low or line dry

Best plant based/natural detergents are:

- Biokleen (not HE safe)
- Method (HE safe)
- Ology
- Kirkland Signature Environmentally Responsible *HE Safe
- Seventh Generation *HE Safe
- Planet
- Sun *HE safe (Free & Clear version)

Ammonia build-up can be very difficult to remove. We have found Rockin' Green's Funk Rock Ammonia Bouncer useful in both removing ammonia as well as for preventive use in the rinse cycle before washing to keep ammonia away.

Plant Based/Natural Detergents that are NOT effective:

- Allen's Naturally
- Molly's Suds
- Ecos
- Nellie's
- Crunchy Clean
- Honest Co
- BumGenius
- Rock n Green
- Soap Nuts
- Eco Nuts
- Soap Berries
- Charlie's Soap
- Country Save
- Ecosprout

Sunlight

For troublesome stains or persistent odor, dry cloth diapers out in the sun for a few hours after washing. The UV rays bleach out the stains and can help kill the odor causing bacteria. Be careful with waterproof lining in hot sun as they can actually melt.

Machine Drying

Keep in mind that occasional machine drying (if an option) can help keep cloth diapers clean by killing bacterial build-up. Avoid drying cloth diapers containing waterproofing, elastic, or Velcro/hook and loop closures on high heat, as this will degrade them much quicker.

Fabric Softener

EWG recommends Green Shield Organic Fabric Softener, Lavender Mint. This is the only one rated an A score on their website.

20

"*TANGLED*" HAIR AND SKIN CARE PRODUCTS

Eat Your Way to Healthy Skin with Food Nutrients

Our skin is the largest organ in our body. Enjoy eating the foods listed below to add nutrients, vitamins, minerals, antioxidants and phytonutrients to improve our skin and overall health.

Vitamin A Foods: Carrots, sweet potato, spinach, swiss chard, kales

Helps: Promote cell turnover, acne, anti-aging, dry skin, eczema

Vitamin C Foods: Oranges, dark leafy greens, papaya, bell peppers, pineapple, strawberries

Helps: Collagen structure, antioxidant, UV protection, dry skin

Vitamin E Foods: Kale, broccoli, spinach, collard greens, brussels sprouts, olive oil

Helps: Anti-inflammatory, UV protective, atopic dermatitis, psoriasis

Omega-3 Fatty Acid Foods: Walnuts, ground chia seeds and flaxseeds, fish oil, sea plants (seaweed)

Helps: anti-inflammatory, moisturizing, acne, psoriasis, dry skin, dermatitis

Probiotics: fermented foods, probiotic supplements, kombucho

Helps: Intestinal health, rosacea, psoriasis, acne, dry skin

Zinc Foods: Cashews, garbanzo beans, sesame and pumkin seeds, asparagus, quinoa

Helps: anti-inflammatory, wound healing, acne, anti-aging

Biotin Foods: Almonds, tomatoes, carrots, onions, oats, sweet potatoes

Helps: skin moisturing, dermatitis, cradle carp, dandruff, hair loss

Sulfur Foods: Kale, garlic, broccoli, onions, legumes, asparagus, brussels sprouts Helps: Collagen production, antioxidant glutathione, anti-inflammatory, anti-again

Thousands of Toxic Chemicals in Skin Care Products

I have used the Environmental Working Group to investigage the thousands of toxic chemicals in hair, skin care, make-up, shampoos, and sunscreens. There are over 97,000 products listed there to show you how many of the products you use every day are toxic. It is a great way to find alternatives and safer products for adults, your babies, and your older kids/teens. The group evaluates thousands of ingredient labels to keep you constantly updated. **An EWG study found that personal care products expose children to an average of 60 chemicals every day that they can breathe in or that absorb through their skin.**

Please go to https://www.ewg.org/skindeep for additional information on all skin care products.

Babies and young children's immature organs are still developing and need to be protected from the world of toxins that are in the majority of personal care products, including baby products. Unfortunately, most of the commercial baby products are not safe and many contain very harmful toxins that can contaminate our babies bodies, leading to disease later in life.

EWG product testing, conducted in partnership with Health Care Without Harm and other members of the Campaign for Safe Cosmetics, showed phthalates in three-quarters of 72 name-brand products tested. The following shows the toxins in products on the left and the best recommended product on the right:

Toxins in Soaps	EWG Best Tested Least Toxic
triclosan and triclocarban	Dr. Desai Soap, LLC
	Lion Bear Naked Soap Co. Most
conventional soap products	Sunfeather Artisan Soap Company

Toxins in Skin moisturizer products	EWG Best Tested Least Toxic
Retinyl palmitate	Beyond Organic Skincare Light 24 Hour Moisturizer for Sensitive Skin)
Retinyl acetate	Conscious Skincare Gentle Day & Night Moisturizer
Retinoic acid	Delizioso Skincare Oil Free Facial Moisturizer, Nettle & Herbs
Retinol in daytime products	

Toxins in Sunscreens	Adult Skin moisturizers with Sunscreen
All Suncreens toxins listed below	100% Pure Healthy Skin Tinted Moisturizer
	DeVita Natural Skin Care Solar Body Moisturizer, SPF 30

EWG Safer & Least Toxic Kids Sunscreens

Wear hats and shade mid day, infants under 6 months should not be in the sun at all or wear sunscreen. The only choice from EWG is **Butterbean Sunscreen Aerosol** (only one rated 1 by EWG)

Toxins in Sunscreens: Oxybenzone, Octinoxate (Octylmethoxycinnamate), Titanium Dioxide, Zinc Oxide, Avobenzone, Mexoryl SX, Retinyl palmitate, spray & powder sunscreen, SPF above 50 (worst)

EWG Best Tested Least Toxic

Jack N' Jill Natural Toothpaste
Davids Natural Toothpaste, Inc.
Cleure Hypoallergenic, Mint Free Toothpaste
Redmond Earthpaste Amazingly Natural Toothpaste
Arganat ALL NATURAL CLAY TOOTHPASTE - NATURE
Daisy Blue Naturals Natural Powder Toothpaste (toothpaste)
Desert Essence Natural Tea Tree Oil & Neem Toothpaste, Wintergreen

Dr. Bronner's Anise All-One Toothpaste
Healthy Home Company Toothpaste
Just the Goods vegan toothpaste
Made Simple Skin Care Mint Sweet Orange Toothpaste
Miessence Anise Toothpaste
Modere Toothpaste REFRESH (toothpaste)
Poofy Organics Happy Teeth Toothpaste
Real Purity Certainly Cinnamon Toothpaste
The Peelu Co. Toothpaste, Peppermint
Tom's of Maine

Avoid: triclosan

EWG Best Tested Least Toxic

Orly
Piggy Paint
Poofy Polish
Acquarella Water Color Girly
Kiss Salon Toenail kit
Rococo Supergloss
Suncoat Girl Natural

Toxins in Nail Polish: Formaldehyde, formalin, hardeners, tolune, dibutyl phthalate (DBP) Pregnant…skip Polish

EWG Best Tested

Dr. Brown's Pacifier and Bottle Wipes, Unscented
WaterWipes Baby Wipes
Babyganics Face, Hand & Baby Wipe Fragrance Free
Babyganics Hand & Face Wipes, Fragrance Free
BabySpa Ultra-Soft Baby Wipes

The Honest Company Honest Wipes
Toxins in baby wipes: Bronopol, DMDM hydantoin, Fragrance

EWG Best Tested Least Toxins

Ava Anderson Non Toxic Baby Diaper Cream
Badger Zinc Oxide Diaper Cream
Belly Buttons & Babies Diaper Cream, Unscented
Desert Essence Don't Be Rash Diaper Cream
Little Twig Organic Diaper Cream, Extra-Mild, Unscented
Penny Lane Organics Happy Baby 100% Natural
Overnight strength Diaper Rash Cream
Sona Organics Diaper Cream
The Honest Company Honest Diaper Rash Cream

Toxins in Diaper Cream: BHA, Boric acid, Fragrance

EWG Best Tested Least Toxic Shampoo

Ava Anderson Non Toxic Baby Body Wash & Shampoo
Aveeno Baby Cleansing Therapy Moisturizing Wash, F F
Babo Botanicals Oatmilk Calendula Moisturizing Baby Shampoo & Wash
Babyganics Shampoo + Body Wash, FF
Beautycounter Baby Gentle All-Over Wash
Belly Buttons & Babies Mom & Baby Body Wash/Shampoo, Unscented
Burt's Bees Baby Bee Shampoo & Wash, Fragrance Free
Beautycounter Kidscounter Nice Do Shampoo
Real Purity Natural & Gentle Baby Shampoo
Enkido Shampoo
Herbal Choice Mari Shampoo, Organic
A Soap for Goodness Sake Babassu Shampoo and Body Bar
Ethiks Shampoo, Face & Body Wash
Morrocco Method Int'l Pine Shale Shampoo Air

Toxins in Baby Shampoos: Retinyl Palmitate, Fragrance, Ceteareth-12, Sulisobenzone, Benzophenone 4, Glycerin, UREA (Cancer), Sodium Laureth Sulfate, Polyquaternium-7, Tocopheryl Acetate, Phytantriol, Peg-120 Methyl glucose dioleate, Phenoxyethanol, Metlparaben, Peg-7 Glyceryl cocoate, BHT (Cancer), Iodopropynyl Butylcarbamate, Ethylhexyl Methoxycinnamate, Octinoxate, Propylparaben

EWG Best Tested and Least Toxins

Primal Life Organics Primal Hair Spray, Sweet
Carina Botanical Therapeutic Tree Essence Natural Hairspray
Carina Pure & Natural Fast Drying Hairspray
Just the Goods vegan leave in hair conditioning spray
Morrocco Method Int'l Agave Mist Styling Spritz & Hair Spray
Professional by Nature's Therapy Volumizing Hairspray, Firm Hold

Toxins in Hair Sprays: Fragrance, Octinoxate, Ethylhexyl methoxycinnamate, Alcohol denatured, lactic acid, sodium lactate, potassium sorbate, Aminomethyl propanol, Sodium benzoate, Urea, Propylene glycol, Pentane, Acrylates/octylacrylamide copolymer, Punica, Punica granatum, Fructose, Glycine, Hydrofluorocarbon 152, Punica granatum (pomegranate) extract, Inositol, Sorbitol, Niacinamine, Punica granatum extract, Piper nigrum (black pepper) seed extract

Make up

Please go to the following site to look up the safer/lower toxic make up for face, eyes and lips including those found in foudations, eye shadows, blushes, eye pencils, concealers, lip glosses, etc.

https://www.ewg.org/skindeep/search.php?query=makeup&h=Search

Stay Away from

Hand sanitizers

Perfume, cologne, and body spray

"Fragrance" in everything

Loose powders

Baby powder - tiny airborne particles can damage baby's delicate, developing lungs

The EWG states "Because federal law contains no safety standard for cosmetics, it is legal for companies to use ingredients that are reproductive toxins like phthalates, carcinogens, and other potentially harmful substances."

Chemicals to Avoid

The average woman uses 12 products containing 168 different ingredients daily. These cosmetic chemicals penetrate into the skin's inner layers, the bodies largest organ. Chemicals found in our bodies include: industrial plasticizers called phthalates; parabens, which are preservatives; and persistent fragrance components like musk xylene.

Alpha and beta hydroxy acids: (lactic acid and glycolic acid) FDA issued a consumer warning that commercial "skin peel" products, advertised to remove wrinkles, blemishes, blotches and acne scars, could destroy the upper layers of the skin, causing severe burns, swelling, and pain. FDA's Office of Women's Health sponsored studies that have linked these ingredients to UV-induced skin damage and potential increased risks of skin cancer.

Hair dye: Minimize use of dark, permanent hair dyes. Many contain coal tar ingredients, including aminophenol, diaminobenzene, and phenylenediamine, linked to cancer.

Skin lighteners: Avoid skin lighteners with hydroquinone. FDA warns that this skin-bleaching chemical can cause a skin disease called ochronosis, with "disfiguring and irreversible" blue-black lesions on exposed skin. Always avoid products with "mercury," "calomel", "mercurio" or "mercurio chloride" which can be in illegal imported skin lighteners.

Avoid keratin treatments: Formaldehyde mixed with water creates a new chemical, methylene glycol. Most keratin treatments that were tested contain formaldehyde even when most advertised they did not.

BHA: The National Toxicology Program classifies butylated hydroxy-anisole (BHA) as "reasonably anticipated to be a human carcinogen." BHA produces liver damage and causes stomach cancers such as papillomas and carcinomas and interferes with normal reproductive system development and thyroid hormone levels.

Boric acid and Sodium borate: These chemicals disrupt hormones and harm the male reproductive system. The cosmetic industry's own safety panel states that these chemicals are unsafe for infants or those with damaged skin, because they can absorb readily into the body. Despite this guidance, boric acid is found in some diaper creams.

Coal tar: hair dyes and other coal tar ingredients (including Aminophenol, Diaminobenzene, Phenylenediamine) and coal tar, a byproduct of coal processing, is a known human carcinogen, according to the National Toxicology Program and the International Agency for Research on Cancer. It is also in many vitamin B supplements.

Formaldehyde: A potent preservative known as a human carcinogen and neurotoxin by the International Agency on Research on Cancer

Fragrance: It is in so many products from face creams, shampoos, deodorants to laundry detergent. Federal law doesn't require companies to list on product labels any of the chemicals in their fragrance mixture. Fragrances are chemicials and can contain hormone disruptors and are among the top 5 allergens in the world.

Lead: A neurotoxin in popular hair dye Grecian Formula 16 and other black hair dyes for men. Lead from hair dyes travels from hair to doorknobs, cabinets and other household items, where children can ingest it.

Methylisothiazolinone, methylchloroisothiazolinone and benzisothiazolinone: Preservatives, used together in personal care products, among the most common irritants, sensitizers and causes of contact allergy.

Nanoparticles: Topical forms of zinc oxide may produce an allergic reaction on skin, including burning, stinging, itching, tingling, hives, trouble breathing, swelling and dark discoloration, according to the National Institutes of Health. Avoid sprays and powders containing these nanoparticles, which could penetrate your lungs and enter your bloodstream.

Oxybenzone: According to the U.S. Centers for Disease Control and Prevention, in human epidemiological studies this sunscreen agent and ultraviolet light absorber is found in the bodies of nearly all Americans. Oxybenzone has been linked to hormone disruption and potentially to cell damage that may lead to skin cancer. **A study of 404 New York City women in the third trimester of pregnancy associated higher maternal concentration of oxybenzone with a decreased birth weight among newborn baby girls but with greater birth weight in newborn boys.** Studies on cells and laboratory animals indicate that oxybenzone may disrupt the hormone system.

Parabens (specifically Propyl-, Isopropyl-, Butyl-, and Isobutyl- parabens): Parabens are estrogen-mimicking preservatives used widely in cosmetics. The CDC has detected parabens in virtually all Americans bodies. According to the European Commission's Scientific Committee on Consumer Products, longer chain parabens like propyl and butyl paraben and their branched counterparts, isopropyl parabens and isobutylparabens, may disrupt the endocrine system and cause reproductive and developmental disorders.

Petroleum distillates: Petroleum-extracted cosmetics ingredients are found in mascara. They may cause contact dermatitis and are often contaminated with cancer-causing impurities. Petroleum for mascara is produced in oil refineries at the same time as automobile and heating fuel.

Phthalates: Industrial chemicals used to soften PVC plastic and a solvents used in cosmetics

- Toys
- Vinyl flooring
- Detergents
- Lubricating oils
- Food packaging
- Pharmaceuticals
- Blood bags and tubing
- Nail polish
- Soaps
- Hair sprays
- Aftershave lotions
- Shampoos
- Perfumes

They can damage the liver, kidneys, lungs, and reproductive system — particularly the developing testes. **Pregnant women should avoid nail polish containing dibutyl phathalate.** Everyone should avoid products with "fragrance" indicating a chemical mixture that may contain phthalates.

Resorcinol: Common ingredient in hair color, personal care products and bleaching products. It can irritate the skin, it is toxic to the immune system and can disrupt normal thyroid function.

Toluene: Volatile petrochemical solvent and paint thinner and potent neurotoxicant that acts as an irritant, impairs breathing, causes nausea and can be toxic to the immune system. **A pregnant woman's exposure to toluene vapors during pregnancy may impair fetal development**. Some evidence suggests a link to malignant lymphoma.

Vitamin A compounds (listed as: retinol, retinyl palmitate, retinyl acetate) in skin and lip products, sunscreens and makeup. Furthermore sun exposture breaks down vitamin A to produce toxic free radicals that can damage DNA and hasten tumors in lab animals.

Animal-based ingredients: Make sure to check websites to see if your products use animal ingredietns or are labeled as "cruelity to animals". Choose products that are labeled with PETA, Vegan, Vegetarian or Leaping Bunny logos.

Triclosan & Triclocarban: is very toxic to the aquatic environment and disrupts thyroid function and reproductive hormones. Use organic approved soaps and water to prevent the spread of infections.

Triclocarban and triclosan in everything listed below

Soap: Dial® Liquid Hand Soap and Body Wash; Tea Tree Therapy™ Liquid Soap; Clearasil® Daily Face Wash; Dermalogica® Skin Purifying Wipes; DermaKleen™ Antibacterial Lotion Soap; CVS Antibacterial Soap; Ajax Antibacterial Dish Soap; Kimcare Antibacterial Clear Soap; Bath and Body Works Antibacterial Hand Soaps; Gels and Foaming Sanitizers

Dental Care: Colgate Total®; Breeze™ Daily Mouthwash; Reach® Antibacterial Toothbrush

Cosmetics: Garden Botanika® Powder Foundation; Mavala Lip Base; Movate® Skin Litening Cream HQ; Paul Mitchell Detangler Comb; Revlon ColorStay LipSHINE Lipcolor Plus Gloss; Babor Volume Mascara; Phytomer Perfect Visage Gentle Cleansing Milk; Phytomer Hydracontinue Instant Moisture Cream, Bath and Body Works Antibacterial Moisturizing Lotions

Deodorant: Arm and Hammer® Essentials Natural Deodorant; Queen Helene® Tea Trea Oil Deodorant and Aloe Deodorant; DeCleor Deodorant Stick; Epoch® Deodorant with Citrisomes

First Aid: SyDERMA® Skin Protectant plus First Aid Antiseptic; Healwell Plantar Fasciitis Night Splint; Solarcaine® First Aid Medicated Spray; Nexcare™ First Aid Skin Crack Care; Universal Cervical Collar with Microban

Kitchenware: Farberware® Microban Cutting Boards; Franklin Machine Products FMP Ice Cream Scoop SZ 20 Microban; Hobart Semi-Automatic Slicer; Chix® Food Service Wipes with Microban; Compact Web Foot® Wet Mop Heads

Other Personal Care Products: Murad Acne Complex® Kit, ®; Diabet-x™ Cream; Scunci Microban Comb; Sportslick Pocket Slick

Clothes: Biofresh® socks; undergarments; tops and bottoms

Office and School Products: Ticonderoga® Pencils with Microban Protection; Avery® Touchgaurd View Binders; C-line® products; Clauss® cutting instruments; Costco® products; Sharp® printing calculators; Westcott® scissors

Other: Bionare® Cool Mist Humidifier; Deciguard AB® Antimicrobial Ear Plugs; Bauer® Re-Akt hockey helmet and 7500 hockey helment; Miller Paint Acro Pure Interior Paint; Holmes Foot Buddy™ HMH120U Antimicrobial

Foot Buddy Foot Warmer; Blue Mountain Wall Coverings, California Paints®; Davis Paint® Perfection; Hirschfield's Paint®,; O'Leary Paint®; EHC AMRail Escalator Handrails, Dupont™ Air Filters; Winix Dehumidifiers; J Cloth® towels; select Quickie cleaning products; Kimberly Clark® WYPALL X80 Towels; Canopy® kitchen towels; ALUF Plastics®; BioEars earplugs; Petmate® LeBistro feeders and waterers; Infantino cart covers and baby carriers; Oreck XL®; Bissell Healthy Home Vacuum™; NuTone® Central Vacuum systems; Rival® Seal-A-Meal® Vacuum Food Sealer; CleenFreek SportsHygiene Yoga Mat; Resilite Sports Products; Rubbermaid® Coolers; Stufitts sports gear; Venture Products® fitness mats; Custom Building Products; DAP®Kwik Seal Plus®; Laticrete; Niasa Biquichamp® mortar grout and sealant; ProAdvanced Products

21

"SLEEPING BEAUTY" HOW TO GET TO SLEEP AND STAY THERE

Mattress – A Bed of Nails

Our babies will spend over 16 hours on their toxic mattress, many times breathing in the dangerous gases from their fire retardant mattresses. The EWA released a study of foam from 20 old and new crib mattresses. They found that "mattresses release up to 30 different types of volatile organic compounds, also known as VOCs, among them, phenol, a strong skin and respiratory irritant. The study detected other chemicals, including linalool and limonene, known fragrance allergens that can cause skin allergies. Repeated exposure over time increases the chances of an allergic reaction".

The EWA produced the study listed above, but no suggestions for safe mattresses were available. Always check the EWG site for updates. This is the safest mattress I could find; however, there may be other safe ones available to look for.

Naturepedic states they are the only company that uses low density, food-grade polyethylene for waterproofing and dust mite proofing. Strict independent testing confirms there are no phthalates or any toxic chemicals in this polyethylene. It also contains no wool, latex or polyurethane foam. They use organic cotton fabric, organic cotton fiber and PLA fiber (made from plant starch). The mattresses pass all Federal and State flammability standards without the use of any fire retardant chemicals or barriers. In a Naturepedic mattress, there are no flame-retardants, no perfluorinated chemicals (PFCs), no antibacterial treatments or biocides, no glues or adhesives, no allergens, and no GMO cotton or other GMO fibers. If you do not want the waterproof plastic covering, they also offer a non-waterproof quilted organic cotton crib mattress with a certified organic cotton covering. The information was taken from the Healthy Child website. https://www.healthychild.com/safe-non-toxic-organic-crib-mattresses/

Don't Forget the Toxins in Furniture

On January 23rd, 2015, the Chicago Tribune reported that major furniture retailers including Crate and Barrel, Room and Board, Williams-Sonoma (Pottery Barn, West Elm) have mostly eliminated chemicals known as toxic flame retardants from their furniture.

Are You a Walking Zombie?

What does Rip Van Winkle and Sleeping beauty have in common? They can sleep....deep sleep, something that 47 percent of the population in the US is not getting. Half of Americans (48%) say they do not get enough sleep, but less than half of them take any specific action to help themselves get better sleep. We walk around as zombies just going through the motions of life. You see them, or maybe this is you....the ones yawning all day, not able to focus, blurred vision, head on the desk, falling asleep watching TV.

Symptoms of sleep deprivation in adults include:

- Constant yawning
- Doze off when sitting still
- Grogginess when waking in the morning
- Sleepy all day long
- Poor concentration and mood changes (more irritable)

Symptoms of Sleep Deprivation in Children

- Speed up instead of slow down
- Moodiness and irritability
- Temper tantrums
- Emotionally explosive at the slightest provocation
- Over-activity and hyperactive behavior
- Daytime naps
- Grogginess when they wake up
- Hard to get out of bed
- Feel angry
- Impulsive
- Mood swings
- Feel sad
- Depressed
- Lack motivation

Sleep Deficiency can Cause Problems

- Learning
- Focusing
- Making decisions
- Solving problems
- Remembering things
- Controlling your emotions
- Behavior
- Coping with change
- Trouble finishing tasks
- Slower reaction time
- Making more mistakes

Sleep Disorder Facts

An estimated 50-70 million US adults have sleep or wakefulness disorder

Snoring is a major indicator of obstructive sleep apnea

The National Department of Transportation estimates drowsy driving to be responsible for 1,550 fatalities and 40,000 nonfatal injuries annually in the United States

More women feel that they are not getting enough sleep (53%) than men (44%)

"Rock a Bye Baby" - How Much Sleep do We Need?

Newborn-2 months (Night) 8 hours plus (Naps) 7-9 hours

2-4 months (Night) 9-10 hours (Naps) 4-5 hours

4-6 months (Night) 14-15 hours (Naps) 4-5 hours
6-9 months (Night) 10-11 hours (Naps) 3-4 hours
9-12 months (Night) 10-12 hours (Naps) 2-3 hours
12-18 months (Night) 11-12 hours (Naps) 1-2 hours
18 months - 2 years (Night) 11 hours (Nap) 2 hours
2-3 years (Night) 10-11 hours (Nap) 1-2 hours
3-5 years (Night) 11-13 hours (Naps) 0-1 hours
5-12 years (Night) 10-11 hours (Naps) 0
Teens 9-10.5 hours
Adults 7-8 hours

The National Institutes of Health suggests that, according to data from the National Health Interview Survey, nearly 30% of adults reported an average of ≤6 hours of sleep per day in 2005-2007.3 In 2009, only 31% of high school students reported getting at least 8 hours of sleep on an average school night.

Three Stages to REM Sleep

We need to make sure we get the recommended amount of sleep to be alert mentally sharp, emotionally balanced, and full of energy all day long. In addition, we need quality sleep, which means at least 20 percent of the night in REM sleep.

Rapid eye movement sleep (REM sleep, REMS) has been defined, as is a unique phase of mammalian sleep characterized by random movement of the eyes, low muscle tone throughout the body, and the propensity of the sleeper to dream vividly. Electrical and chemical activity regulating this phase seems to originate in the brain stem and is characterized most notably by an abundance of the neurotransmitter acetylcholine, combined with a nearly complete absence of monoamine neurotransmitters histamine, serotonin, and norepinephrine.

Stage 1 – Wakefulness, easy to wake up, your eyes are closed 5 – 10 minutes' in.

Stage 2 – Non Rapid Eye Movement - light sleep. Your heart rate slows and your body temperature drops.

Stage 3 – Rapid Eye Movement – REM sleep, deep sleep stage, harder to wake, the body repairs and regrows tissues, builds bone and muscle, and strengthens the immune system. 90 minutes after you fall asleep, heart rate and breathing quickens, more intense dreams, brain is more active.

BABIES get up to 50 percent of their sleep in REM sleep.

Daytime Helpful Hints

- Wake up with sunlight: take a walk outside, sit on your deck with your coffee, park far away from your office to expose yourself to bright sunlight. Your eyes need 10 minutes of sunlight everyday so leave your sunglasses off.
- Keep your curtains open and let as much natural light into your home or office.
- Exercise during the day, even a ten-minute walk helps. Sleep speeds up your metabolism, elevates body temperature, and stimulates activating hormones such as cortisol. It takes about 6 hours for the body to fully cool down after exercising to a temperature conducive to sleep.
- It is recommended to drink no more than one 8 oz. cup of organic coffee in the morning per day. Do not consume sodas or any other product with caffeine. Caffeine can keep us awake up to ten to twelve hours after drinking it.
- Do meditation once or twice a day to help de-stress. Meditation helps get rid of what's on our mind from stress to our daily to do list.
- Mix 1 tsp. with at least 28 oz. of water of Premiers Max B (for adults only) and drink all day.

Catch some zzzzz's - Nighttime

- Got to bed at the same time every night and get up at the same time
- Do not drink alcohol as it interferes with your sleep process. You may fall asleep but it interferes with your body's natural rhythm and many will wake up in the night, especially to use the bathroom.

- Do not use computers, phones, tablets, any type of technology at least one to two hours before bed. The blue light emitted by electronics is especially disruptive. Try turning the brightness down, or using light-altering software such as flux that adjusts the color of your display. Your body needs to detox from the EMF that is transmitting through your body.
- Say no to late night television
- Minimize the time that you stay up later or sleep in as it will disrupt your internal clock.
- If you need a nap during the day make sure you do not sleep more than 20 minutes.
- Do not fall asleep early on the couch. Get up and do something mildly stimulating to distract you so you can fall asleep at your normal time.
- Do not have lights or a television on when you are going to sleep.
- Melatonin is a naturally occurring hormone controlled by light exposure that helps regulate your sleep-wake cycle. Your brain secretes more melatonin when it is dark—making you sleepy—and less when it is light—making you more alert. However, many aspects of modern life can alter your body's natural production of melatonin and shift your natural body clock rhythm.

Right Before Bed

1. Listen to soothing music or nature sounds, read a real book, Nook Glowlight or listen to an audio books
2. Make sure the room is dark, cool and quiet
3. Move digital clock at least 6 feet from where you sleep
4. Take Melatonin or Tranquiol (Premier Research Lab) 1 hour before bed
5. Wear a sleep mask
6. Rub essential oils, especially lavender, between your hands and inhale
7. Take a hot bath or shower before bed
8. If you do get up, do not turn a light on, instead have a nightlight on.
9. Relax in the evening, do not exercise before bed, it revs up your metabolism

10. Do yoga or gentle stretching before bed
11. Avoid drinking lots of liquids before bed
12. Stop eating two hours before bedtime. Meats take a long time to digest so keep them for your dinner meal. Snacks can include a fruit, especially bananas or raw nuts, something small and easier to digest.
13. Sleep with earplugs, but not if you have children, you need to listen for.
14. Make sure your bed and pillow is comfortable. Do not go cheap when buying a mattress or pillow.
15. Have sex before bedtime – produces serotonin and relaxation.
16. Close your eye, take slow, deep breathes and imagine you are at your favorite peaceful place (beach).
17. Progressive muscle relaxation. Starting with your toes, tense all the muscles as tightly as you can one at a time until you finish with your neck. Then completely relax.
18. If you wake and cannot get back to sleep, write down what is bothering you or make a "to-do list" for the next day with a dim light. Go down on the floor and do yoga stretches. Get back in bed and do the progressive relaxation and deep breathing.

Sleep Apnea

The most common signs of obstructive sleep apnea are loud and chronic snoring, which includes, gasping for air and sometimes choking. The snoring usually is loudest when you sleep on your back. Another symptom is being sleepy all day.

Signs and Symptoms of Sleep Apnea Include

- Snoring
- Sleepy during the day
- Morning headaches
- Memory or learning problems and not being able to concentrate
- Feeling irritable, depressed, or having mood swings or personality changes
- Waking up frequently to urinate
- Breathe through mouth
- Dry mouth or sore throat when you wake up

Children can also have sleep apnea. It can cause hyperactivity, poor school performance, and angry or hostile behavior. Children who have sleep apnea also may breathe through their mouths instead of their noses during the day.

22

"TOY STORY" - SAFETY, LEARNING, BAD PLASTIC

There are so many things to worry about when it comes to the safety of our children. Everyone with a new infant/child should be well acquainted with the United States Consumer Product Safety Commission, the World Against Toys Causing Harm (WATCH), and Kidshealth.org. I have listed the information below if you need to contact them or just like to be up to date with the most current recalls. The few I listed below are just the most recent recalls from Jan/Feb 2016 to show you the variety of different items that may pose a danger to your child.

1. United States Consumer Product Safety Commission
   Phone: (301) 504-7923
   Hours: M-F 8 a.m. - 4:30 p.m. ET
   Fax: (301) 504-0124 and (301) 504-0025
   http://www.cpsc.gov/en/About-CPSC/Contact-Information/
   Toll-Free Consumer Hotline: Phone: (800) 638-2772; TTY (301) 595-7054
   Hours: Mon.-Fri. 8 a.m. to 5:30 p.m.; messages can be left anytime.

2. World Against Toys Causing Harm (WATCH)
   A non-profit organization dedicated to educating the public about dangerous children's products and protecting children from harm.
   http://toysafety.org/ |watch@toysafety.org Phone: (617) 723-6511

Nuna Baby Essentials Recalls High Chairs Due to Fall Hazard: The arm bar can bend or detach during use, posing a fall hazard to children.

KHS America Recalls Children's Musical Instrument Due to Violation of Lead Paint Standard Hazard: The pink metal note bar on the glockenspiel may contain excessive levels of lead in the paint, violating the federal lead paint standard. If the paint is scraped off and ingested, lead can cause adverse health effects.

Wedgwood Decorative Baby Rattles Recalled by WWRD Due to Choking Hazard: The ball bearings inside each side of the decorative rattle can be released, posing a choking hazard to young children

Chillafish Recalls Children's Balance Bikes Due to Laceration Hazard (Recall Alert): Overinflated tires can cause the wheel rims to crack and send pieces of the plastic rim flying, posing a laceration hazard to consumers.

Britax Recalls Strollers and Replacement Top Seats Due to Choking Hazard: The foam padding on the stroller's arm bar can come off in fragments if the child bites the arm bar, posing a choking hazard.

If we are lucky, a new product that is recalled will be on the news or taken off before we even purchase it. However, be careful when you are purchasing used toys, hand me downs, or items from a garage sale. You may be buying a product that is on the recall list. It is important that parents constantly educate themselves about these dangerous toys.

"I Don't Want to Grow Up ...I'm a Toys R Us Kid" – Keep Your Kids Safe

1. Babies love to put objects into their mouths so avoid any toy with parts that can come apart, and especially balls less than 1.75 inches in diameter. Small parts can become lodged in the windpipe
2. Watch for toys with long handles, babies can put these handles in their mouths and can choke themselves
3. Avoid battery-operated toys for babies, since battery acid could leak and be ingested by the child or they can swallow the battery. If the toy does have a battery, ensure the battery compartment is secured and is not easily accessible by your infant.

4. Watch out for any toy with a string longer than six inches, especially pull toys. These strings can pose a strangulation hazard
5. Do not use crib toys that hang down from or across the crib, since these can entrap a child or present a strangulation hazard
6. Check to make sure any painted toy uses lead-free paint, since lead exposure can lead to serious developmental delays
7. Watch out for any riding toy that does not have a harness or that is not labeled for use by babies
8. Do not use toys with small holes in them that can harbor mold, especially bath toys that absorb water
9. Do not purchase any toys that have BPA in them

Age Birth to 6 months

In the beginning months, our babies will be more interested in sounds (music), vision (bright colors), movement (mobiles) or a toy they can grab at or kick at.

1. A crib mobile is a great way to attract all the senses, where your baby can watch lights, relax to music and grab at things in front of them. I would only suggest mobiles that can be used only in your presence. If you choose mobiles for a crib, make sure there are no strings attached that could cause strangulation.
2. Baby's vision is limited so books with large images are great to introduce to a young baby. Babies enjoy listening to your voice while you are reading or even singing to them. Purchase books with large images, very colorful and different patterns.
3. Hand held rattles and soft toys can spark an array of sensory experiences. Rattles will amuse your baby and help strengthen motor abilities.
4. Floor mats make for a creative playtime and a different position for babies with colorful pictures, sounds and things to grab at. Babies start to roll over between 2 and 6 months.
5. Mirrors are also great since babies are drawn to faces and other parts of their bodies like feet and hands.

Age 6 months to a Year

Babies are ready to learn even before they are born forming connections through stimulation with sight, sound, touch, taste and smell. The more you challenge your child with a variety of experiences, the more advanced your baby's sensory and motor development will be. This period is great for interactive play.

1. Babies will start to watch large images on television. This may be a good time to introduce educational videos and music to stimulate their hearing and vision.
2. Babies will start to develop their hand-eye coordination by clapping their hands and waving. They also start to crawl, rock back and forth, and walk. They begin to make sounds and single words together. This is a good time for walkers and jumpers to help strengthen their legs to get them ready for walking.
3. This is a great time to purchase toys that make noise, create movement, such as a push, and pull toy.
4. Toys that rock and bounce will help to satisfy their craving for motion.
5. Books will become more interesting and should be read on a daily basis.
6. Although kids today are interested in internet games, it is best to limit their exposure to the effects of not only electromagnetic fields but also they will lose interest in the other developmental games.

12 - 18 Months

By now, most babies are toddlers and have discovered the world in an upright position. They begin to walk, climb and jump. They require more activity. It is important to embrace this but at the same time to encourage focus with a continuation of education learning toys. Kids start to explore, and get into trouble with dangerous situations at this age, requiring attention that is a lot more direct and include intervention. Toddlers seem to be more goal oriented, and learn mostly through imitating others including adults and other children.

1. Toys requiring more motor skills such as puzzles, building blocks, reading, shapes, colors and numbers
2. Outside activities such as riding a trike, running outside, sliding down a slide, swinging, throwing balls, hide and seek
3. Introducing musical instruments such as pianos, guitars, and drums
4. Educational games on the internet, television and games (limit)

18 - 24 Months

Children really start to use their imagination and make believe. This is a critical time as toddlers learn to problem solve and figure things out on their own. They are now at an age where they can start to follow simple instructions. This is a time to really encourage them to help you pick up their toys and start good habits. They also begin to identify colors, numbers, verbally count, and match objects by color and shape. It is such a great time to enjoy your child's fast-paced vocabulary, sometimes learning several new words daily.

1. Riding tricycles, swinging, sliding, rocking horse, riding toys, forts, playhouses
2. Pretending with dolls, action figures, costumes, puppets, kitchen sets, tool sets
3. Music, dancing, playing instruments
4. Stuffed animals
5. Increased reading time

24 - 36 Months

Kids are now ready to be introduced to the world of arts & crafts and board games to really develop their fine motor coordination. This is a great time to start with sports and outdoor games. Children will always need to have special time devoted for learning through games, books and projects.

1. Painting and coloring (use of crayons, chalk and paint)
2. Working with clays
3. Cars, trucks and train sets
4. Simple board games
5. Outdoor fun time
6. Imagination toys
7. Work books to introduce phonics, alphabet and numbers

Dangers with Plastic Bath Toys

Dr. Oz just featured a story proving the dangerous problems with mold growing inside your children's baby toys. Make sure that any toy being used does not have any opening where water can seep into it. An inspector featured on the show, cut open a plastic toy to find a large amount of mold growing inside. This can be very dangerous since very young kids suck and chew on their toys.

Phthalates – Toxins Hidden in Your Baby's Plastic

If you are a parent of a young child or are expecting a baby, you need to know about the danger of using phthalates. Phthalates are a group of chemicals used to soften and increase the flexibility of plastic. Phthalates are used in hundreds of consumer products especially pacifiers, teethers and baby bottle nipples, where your baby or child will ingest toxins by simply sucking on these products.

Avoid BPA and Phthalates in the following Items

Toys	Teethers and Baby Nipples	Shampoo, Soap, Lotion	Pacifiers and Rattles	Baby Bottles Sippy Cups
Cleaning Products	Plastic Container	Non Stick Cookware	Plastic Wrap Baggies	Napkins and Toilet Paper
Rubber Ducks	Water Bottles	Plastic Plates	Bath Books	Canned Goods

Tips to minimize exposure to BPA and Phthalates

- Never use plastic containers in microwaves for food or liquids
- Use glass, porcelain and stainless-steel containers for food and beverages, especially hot products
- Only buy plastic, which is BPA Free. If it is not labeled BPA free, look at the bottom of the container and only buy it if it is marked with a 2,4, or 5
- Purchase glass baby bottles for infants or BPA free plastic

FDA States the following with BPA

Here is information for consumers who want to limit their exposure to BPA:

- Plastic containers have recycle codes on the bottom. Some, but not all plastics that are marked with recycle codes 3,6 or 7 may be made with BPA.
- Do not put very hot or boiling liquid that you intend to consume in plastic containers made with BPA. BPA levels rise in food when containers/products made with the chemical are heated and come in contact with the food.
- Discard all bottles with scratches, as these may harbor bacteria and, if BPA-containing, lead to greater release of BPA.

Here is a more recent update for BPA use in packaging for infant formula.

"The U.S. Food and Drug Administration (FDA) will publish a final rule amending the food additive regulations to no longer provide for the use of bisphenol A (BPA)-based epoxy resins as coatings in infant formula packaging because this use has been abandoned."

"The final rule amends 21 CFR 175.300 **to no longer provide for the use of BPA-based epoxy resins as coatings in infant formula packaging.** This rule is effective July 12, 2013. Interested parties may submit objections and requests for a hearing within 30 days of the rule's effective date."

I find it very interesting that the FDA states they are removing the BPA from infant formula packaging, but they are not doing it for safety purposes. Think about everything you buy that is plastic. If it does not say BPA free then it is not. Have you ever driven up to a gas station and notice the cases of water in plastic bottles sitting outside in the sun? Many products today are sent to warehouses that are not temperature regulated. Catch my drift? Maybe it is not such a good idea to drink chemical filled bottled water unless it states it is BPA free.

Read this statement taken directly from the FDA on BPA. The article states they do not feel BPA is a danger, especially to infants, however, they do state the following: Read the entire article at the following link: http://www.fda.gov/forconsumers/consumerupdates/ucm297954.htm.

23

"BEAUTY AND THE BEAST" HORMONE BALANCE

Hormone balance is not easy and many women are affected by nasty symptoms from an early age with the onset of our periods including PMS, painful cramps, and irritability. With a lifetime of toxicity adding to our already mineral and vitamin deficient bodies, we are a hot mess. During pregnancy, the estrogen and progesterone hormones surge as our babies grow. This in turn can trigger cravings (like pickles and ice cream), bloating and mood swings.

On the next page, you will see a chart that identifies all of the hormones in our body. Both men and women have these hormones, so you will see how important each one is and what their jobs are. This is why it is so hard to get the right mix of hormones to get us back on track. Hormone imbalance also affects men and they will most likely need support with testosterone.

Thyroid

The thyroid is one of the most challenging hormones to balance and the estimate is that 1 out of every 5 Americans have a thyroid issue. When the thyroid is not producing the right amount of hormones, many will feel depressed, have low energy, cold hands and feet, and gain weight. since I have seen over 200 people in my practice, I have found that 1 out of every 2 women tested have a thyroid issue. Of course most of my practice consists of women age 45 -55, however these days I am finding many younger women with this issue. If you go to your doctor to get bloodwork for thyroid you will need a Thyroid-Stimulating Hormone (TSH) to test for

Total thyroxine (T4), free thyroxine (FTI or FT4) and Triiodothyronine (T3).

It is important to screen newborns to find out if their thyroid gland function is normal. A condition called congenital hypothyroidism can prevent normal growth and development and can also cause intellectual disability.

QRA Testing for Thyroid

Here's the thing, many tests will not show you have a thyroid issue. I know my thyroid was off since my twenties. It did not show up in a test until late 50's. The QRA test or kinesiology is the only way to see what is going on with your thyroid. You will need to find someone in your area to help you with your thyroid function. I still use Xenostat from Premier as nutrient and enzymes support and my numbers have reversed to normal.

The QRA testing can test all of the hormonal areas. Some women may only need one supplement and others may need a combination of several for balance. Remember that QRA will find a malfunctioning thyroid issue many years before a doctor can find it in a blood test. When a doctor finds it, the thyroid has usually deteriorated to an exhausted state. It can still be brought back to life with the proper nutrition, nutritional supplements and detoxing. The most important supplements for your thyroid are going to be Premiers Xenostat and Thyroven. Make sure to get your thyroid tested to determine which supplements are best to bring you and your thyroid back to life. Also, eating radishes has been known to help balance the thyroid, so pack them into your salads or even better, juice them.

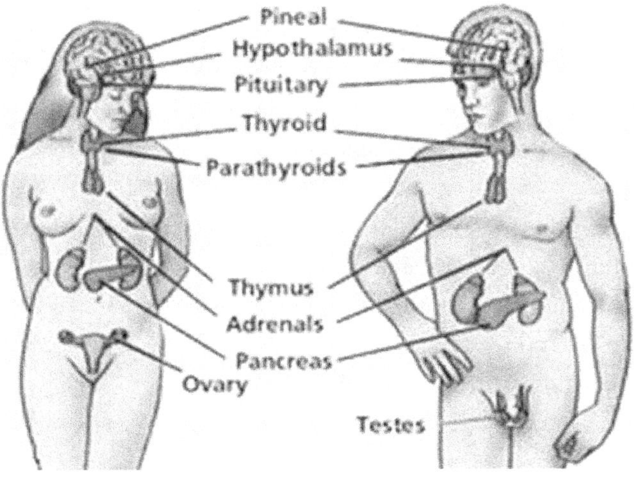

Moans, Groans, Stones, and Bones

If you have any of the symptoms below you may have a hormone imbalance

Loss of energy
Lazy, Lethargic
Tired all the time
Chronic fatigue
Just do not feel well
Do not feel normal
Feel old
Can't concentrate
Depression
Osteoporosis and Osteopenia
Bones hurt: legs and arms
Wake up in middle of night
Trouble getting to sleep
Tired during the day
Irritable and cranky
Forget simple things
Gastric acid reflux
Heartburn; GERD
Decrease in sex drive
Thinning hair
Kidney stones
High Blood Pressure
Recurrent Headaches
Heart Palpitations (arrhythmias)

All These Hormones – No Wonder It is Hard to Balance Them

Estrogens are produced in the ovaries, placenta, liver, adrenals, fat and cells. Their function is for female development, menstruation, pregnancy, and anti-aging.

Pregnenolone is produced in the adrenals. It is responsible for memory and stress resistance.

Cortisol is produced in the adrenals. It is responsible for stress, energy production, mood stability and inflammatory responses.

Vitamin D is produced in the skin, liver and kidneys. It is responsible for muscle, bone and heart health, immunity, cell communication and brain development.

Human Growth Hormone (HGH) is produced in the placenta. It promotes growth in children and adolescents and helps regulate body composition, tissue growth and metabolism in adults.

Melatonin is produced in the pineal gland. It helps promote sleep, supports brain health, heart health, and immune system.

Glucagon is produced in the pancreas. It signals glucose to be transferred to the blood into your cells for energy usage and fat body regulation. It also signals the liver to release glucose into your blood.

Parathyroid Hormone is produced in the parathyroid gland. It controls the amount of calcium in your blood and bones.

Adrenalin is produced in the adrenals. It regulates heart rate, releases glucose and dilates blood vessels.

Thyroid hormone is produced in the thyroid gland. It is responsible for organ development and metabolism.

Progesterone is produced in the ovaries, placenta and the Central Nervous System (CNS.) It is responsible for breast development, female sexual development, menstruation and pregnancy.

Testosterone is produced in the testes and ovaries. They are responsible for male sexual development, sex drive, sperm production and bone and muscle mass.

DHEA is produced in the adrenals and brain. They are responsible for lean body mass, heart health, and resistance to stress.

Ghrelin is produced in the stomach and pancreas. Its job is for fat regulation and to stimulate hunger. Ghrelin is a little gremlin in your stomach that makes you want to tear into some food. Just remember, "Don't Feed Them after Midnight," this little hunger hormone sends messages and travels to your brain and impacts your desire to eat. If you have major food cravings you most likely have a malfunctioning ghrelin. The more you crave sugar, high calorie foods and carbohydrates, the greater your problem. It can also cause a subconscious desire to binge eat or stuff yourself to give you a pleasurable feeling of fullness or satisfaction. Ghrelin activation is vital to maintain your blood sugar during calorie restriction or starvation.

Leptin is produced in the fat cells. It controls fat regulation. Most people that are overweight suffer from a leptin resistance, where it perceives a false state of starvation. This is very important because it activates the ghrelin even if we are full and confuses our metabolism.

Supplements for Pregnancy

For women who are pregnant, or considering pregnancy, the following supplements are suggested for great hormone balance. You will need to be tested with QRA to find out which supplements your body really needs.

Adaptogen-R3

Adaptogens are certain herbs particularly helpful in restoring and maintaining positive homeostasis, the body's natural ability to balance internal and external stress. Adaptogen-R3 is very helpful in supporting hormone balance, hot flashes, weight gain and night sweats. Adaptogen-R3™ contains Nopal cactus, Fo Ti, Rhodiola Rosea and Ecklonia Cava, an invigorating formula that promotes the entire adaptogenic process, including whole body rejuvenation.

UltraPollen

UltraPollen™ is made from premier quality, multiple flower pollen extracts (300 mg/cap) that are 100% allergen and pesticide free (mold spore removed). This premier formula delivers extraordinary flower pollen-based support for health and wellness. UltraPollen is our first choice for those who want to achieve hormone balance. Symptoms of hormone imbalance include a diet high in refined food and a body burden of toxic pesticides/plastic residues.

Colostrum

Colostrum is a special immune-active fluid secreted by a female cow for about three days after giving birth. Our colostrum is obtained from a very select group of dairy farmers dedicated to producing quality colostrum. During the summer, spring and fall, their cows are grass-fed (a superior nutrition source for cattle). During the winter, they are fed hay. This premier quality colostrum passes the U.S.P. pesticide testing. Colostrum-IgG™ is made from bovine colostrum that typically contains 25% immunoglobulins (IgG) (300 mg/tsp, 88 mg/cap) for effective immune support.

EPA/DHA

This distinctive oil blend, which includes the use of flaxseed oil, is a premier quality life-essential fatty acid formula for optimal brain and body support, featuring an ideal blend A (gamma linolenic acid) and Omega 3, 6 and 9 essential fatty acids. Premier EFA Oil Blend is comprised of cold-pressed, premier, unrefined oils that are nitrogen-flushed to protect freshness. This blend has a full-bodied gourmet taste that is delicious mixed in food or drinks. This is important for all kids, adults and especially for pregnant women.

DHA

DHA is an essential plant-source that is derived from non-GMO micro-algae instead of fish, making it suitable for everyone including vegetarians and vegans. Feed your brain with plant-source DHA (docosahexaenoic acid), a key Omega-3 fatty acid, important for digestion. This is most important for ADHD/ADD, Autism, Asthma and all children with any health issues.

Max B

Max B is my favorite and I take it every day. Many of my clients can feel instant energy from our Max B. The liquid form ensures quick delivery and absorption. Our cells prefer Max B's live source, high energy, end-chain vitamin B forms, over common synthetic (coal tar-derived) sources. This B vitamin-rich formula offers advanced support for the liver, energy, immune system, adrenals and mood balance. Carbohydrates can cause vitamin B deficiencies. Problems associated with B vitamin deficiencies include depression, memory loss, heart disease, insomnia, cataracts, atherosclerosis, fatigue, muscle cramps, allergies and GI symptoms to name just a few. This is great for adults, pregnant women and teens.

D3

A one-of-a-kind, live-source vitamin D3 delivers cardiovascular and immune system support. Vitamin D3 also aids in calcium absorption for healthy bones and teeth. Recent studies propose ideal vitamin D3 intake should be 2000 IU or more daily (a recommendation our serum meets in just one drop). Premiers D3 is made with extra virgin olive oil. Kids, teens and adults all need D3, especially if they are not in the sun.

Pink Sea Salt

Premiers pink sea salt is Unrefined, untreated and unheated. Extract from Mediterranean and Hawaiian sea and is rich in trace minerals that children need. A little sea salt each day is a helpful additive for kids, adults, teens and pregnant moms for healthy digestion. ¼ to ½ tsp is a helpful daily dose, without the use of white iodized salt, which a dangerous chemical added to many fast and processed foods.

24
"RAIN RAIN GO AWAY" CHILDREN'S ADDICTION & DEPRESSION

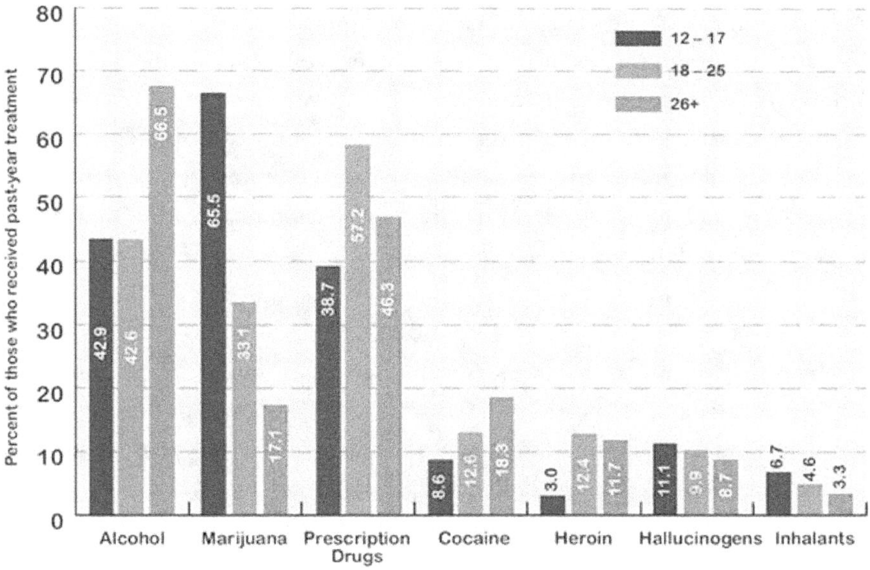

The chart above shows the staggering statistics per age group that are getting treatment for illegal and legal drugs. Children 12-17 are being treated mostly for Marijuana, alcohol and then prescription drugs. The prescription drug use is almost as high as alcohol, which I find especially troubling. This means doctors are prescribing drugs to children at a very young age. We already know alcohol is the mainstream for drug use since it is legal, but I see there is a huge jump in marijuana as well as the prescription drugs.

Over half million Americans die each year from alcohol and tobacco. Over 120 Americans overdose every day from Opiates. Illegal or legal.... "America we have a problem."

What is Addiction & Depression?

To understand addiction and depression we must first understand neurotransmitters in the brain. The neurotransmitters, dopamine and serotonin are responsible for the way we feel, think and act. Scientists have found a genetic link common in people who use drugs, alcohol, chocolate, nicotine, relationships, sex, gambling and any "reward" to make themselves feel better. Addiction can be described as having a dopamine deficiency, which leads to negative emotions, causing a person to seek out stimulating behavior to temporarily increase the dopamine level. Research has shown that successful treatment of addiction requires an understanding of how addictive substances elevate dopamine and serotonin levels in the brain. New "cutting edge" approaches to raising these levels naturally are helping with the intervention and treatment of drug addiction.

Dopamine

When people experience a pleasurable situation, dopamine releases from these nerve cells and is sucked away shortly after by target pumps. However, when drugs enter the brain, they block these pumps leaving the dopamine to swirl around between nerve cells creating a longer lasting high.

The dopamine deficiency experts are calling this the Reward Deficiency Syndrome (RDS). RDS involves the dopamine receptor allele (A1), which reduces dopamine available to the brain. This chemical imbalance blocks the brain's perception of reward. People with this deficiency may feel negative, angry, stressed or depressed much of the time. This is why they turn to

- Drinking
- Drugging
- Smoking
- Gambling

- Shopping
- Sex
- Eating chocolate
- Eating carbohydrates
- Sugar
- Seeking thrills
- Destructive relationships (passion, romance)
- Working addictions
- Computer addictions

Dopamine is associated with feelings of elation, pleasure, satisfaction and reward, which are why a Chemically Dependent Person (CDP) craves the "high". The CDP may inherit the inability to produce enough dopamine. The so-called "lows" a CDP feels may result from the brain's effort to reduce the number of sites that dopamine can connect to. In addition to this, a CDP who continues to use drugs and ingests unhealthy foods will destroy even more dopamine sites. This process fools the brain and slows down the cell production of the neurotransmitters, which causes depression, anxiety and insomnia. Studies show that drugs such as heroin, amphetamine, nicotine and cocaine trigger the release of dopamine that overwhelm the dopamine breakdown process and give them the pleasure they are lacking to start with.

Dopamine activates the body and promotes alertness and energy. There are several ways to increase dopamine naturally in the brain. They include proper nutrition, exercise, supplements and alternative therapies. It is important for a CDP to eat a well-balanced diet consisting of six small meals containing wholesome, whole-grained unprocessed foods. There is a period between meals when the blood sugar levels drop and a person loses energy; a CDP will relapse more often during these low periods. It is also easier for the body to digest and absorb small amounts of food. A sensible choice is plenty of fresh vegetables, fruits, proteins and limited breads and fatty foods.

Exercise is one of the most powerful natural antidepressants we can tap into. It increases endorphins in the brain by raising dopamine for energy. This first became popular in the seventies when runners experienced a rush of good feelings simply called "runners high". Many studies show cardiovascular exercise and weight lifting strongly reduces symptoms of anxiety, depression and low spirits. People that exercise feel better about themselves and have a higher sense of self-esteem. Furthermore, if people transform on the outside they are bound to feel the effects on the inside. So exercise has a biological and psychological effect on the way we feel.

Supplements are natural food derivatives that contribute to the elevation of dopamine. There are numerous supplements that give us energy naturally. My favorite "go to" is Premier Research Labs' Max B. "I don't leave home without it." People with addiction usually have low vitamin B levels.

Alternative Therapies that Increase Dopamine & Serotonin

- Acupuncture
- Acupressure
- Massage
- Chiropractic
- Yoga
- Meditation
- New age music
- Deep breathing
- Walking outside
- Tai Chi
- Exercise

Serotonin

Serotonin has many important brain functions. It gives us a feeling of tranquility, relaxation and calm. A serotonin deficit is believed to be associated with depression, sleep disorders, obesity, violent behavior, PMS and addiction. Serotonin levels are increased by the intake of addictive substances such as alcohol, tobacco, certain narcotics and caffeine.

Serotonin is made from amino acids, which are available when your body digests protein. There are many ways to raise serotonin naturally by either eating, alternative relaxation therapies, or by taking supplements. If a person prefers to eat their way to relaxation, it is recommended to eat foods high in typtophan such as bananas. Current research suggests that sugar and starches are also tranquilizing and promote relaxation, however this is not a healthy way to get there. This is probably why there are so many people that are addicted to sweets and carbohydrates otherwise known as "carb junkies." This approach does not include candies, cakes and fat-laden sweets as they delay the relaxation effect due to their high content of fat.

Supplements Used for Relaxation (Never drive when using these)

My favorite is Tranquinol from Premier Research Labs. I have used this to relax before bedtime when I was unable to sleep. Premier's melatonin is also great for relaxation and successful sleep. Lavender, Stone Root, Valerian, Skullcap, Passion Flower and Oat Straw are also helpful in promoting relaxation.

Students that are struggling with school work often feel badly about themselves. In my study skills group, when I asked the students why they thought they were struggling in school, each replied because "I'm stupid." However, when I explained that they were having difficulty not because they were stupid, but because they did not know there were different ways of learning. They perked up and were motivated to identify their learning style and try new strategies. See more in Chapter 4.

For more information on Addiction, please look forward to my next book which will cover Depression and Addictions.

25

"THE WONDERFUL WORLD OF AHHH" DETOXING

If you are not pregnant yet, or have already had your family, a good detox program can help detox the toxins out of your body. If you are pregnant, you will not be able to do a detox program; just eating healthy foods suggested in this book. I am living proof since I healed from 18 diseases/disorders by detoxing. Detoxing is the complete process that will transform your health to the healthiest you want to be. It is an ongoing process and will depend on how much you are willing to put into it. If you have ever been really ill, especially those who have been for a long time, you know if you don't have your health, you have nothing. "Health is not appreciated until sickness appears."

What is a toxin and Why do I Need to Detox?

Simply put, a toxin is poison to the human body. We can breathe in toxins (from paint, hair spray, smoke), eat toxins (pesticides, antibiotics), drink toxins (BPA in water, sugar, corn syrup), apply toxins (chemicals absorbed through the skin), and inject toxins through vaccines (chemicals injected directly into the blood stream). The human body is amazing as it can self-repair itself, rebuild tissue and replace cells up to a point. It continues to clean up the toxins and get rid of waste by the detox organs listed later in this chapter, until there becomes a huge build up or overload of toxicity. This is when disease starts to set up shop in the body, growing until it gets your attention. This is when we need to start a detox program and eliminate this overload of toxins.

Detoxing is a Three Step Process

First Detoxification - Diet Changes

The first type of detoxing is just changing your diet. You will need to eliminate all toxic foods and drinks from your diet including fast foods, processed foods, white flour & sugar products, dairy and foods containing a lot of chemicals (non-organic foods) from your diet. This will automatically throw your body into a detoxification process. When you add in healthy foods and clean water, your body will start to rid itself of toxins that have been wreaking havoc on your body, causing disease, inflammation, allergies, infections, intolerances, disorders and illness.

Second Detoxification - A Healthy Supplement Program

The second type of detox system is implementing a supplement program. It will nourish your body, giving you and your organs the support they need to start to transform your health. With the deficiency in our soils today, the vitamins and minerals have been depleted, so even if you try to eat well, it is just not enough. If you have abused your body with toxins such as; fast food, processed food, stress, alcohol and drugs, etc., your body is so depleted and hungry for nutrients, enzymes and minerals. The supplements you choose need to meet the following ten requirements:

- Organic
- In a BPA free container
- In a dark colored bottle to block light frequencies
- Liquid supplements or vegetable capsules only (most tablets digest as food)
- No magnesium stearate
- No undesirable oil
- No excipients – fillers and binders
- Animal products organic & humanly treated
- Made from all live sources (plants)
- No synthetic products

If you are currently using supplements and feel no better, know that your supplements do not carry a strong nutritional value of vitamins, minerals and enzymes necessary to really change your health.

Third - Removing the Toxins from Your Body

This is a very important process to help get the toxins out of your body. If you do not have an exit plan, toxins will be released into the bloodstream only to be reabsorbed into the body. You will need to work some of these detoxing techniques into your daily life. The sicker/toxic you are, the more detoxing techniques you will need to use. The more detoxing you do, the faster you will heal.

- Infrared Sauna is a first choice, a healthier and more comfortable
- way to sweat it out than lava rock saunas.
- Purchase an Earthwrappe - infrared heating pad from (Premier Research Labs)
- Soak in a tub with Epsom Salts (health stores or Medi Body Bath by Premier Research Labs)
- Castor Oil Pack (purchase from health food store or Premier Research Labs)
- Dry Skin Brushing (health food stores) to detox the skin
- Liver/Gallbladder flush – purchase from (health store or Premier Research Labs)
- Ionic foot soak (find a health facility that offers this, it releases toxins
- from your feet)
- Do a home foot soak (Premiers Medi Body Bath or Dr. Jernigans Mustard Foot Bath)
- Lymphatic Massage – helps release cogged up toxins from lymph nodes
- Colon Hydrotherapy – find a local health care provider
- Organic Coffee Enemas – (health food stores or Premier Research Labs; will include directions, enema bucket and coffee)
- Exercise and Yoga -moving and stretching your body to eliminate toxins
- Chiropractic - detoxing muscles, bones, tendons, tissue
- QRA with a qualified practitioner. You will need to find a QRA practitioner to start your detox program. The number for Premier Research Labs is (800) 325-7734; they can assist in finding a practitioner in your area
- Emotional detoxing through counseling, hypnosis and de-stressing

How to do a Castor Oil Pack

I use Premier's Castor Oil and Organic Cotton along with my Earthwrappe. The Earthwrappe is important because it's job is to pull toxins out of the body via the infrared system. The great part about the castor oil packs is that you can do them in the privacy of your own home. Here are the instructions for use:

1. Place your organic cotton in a glass bowl and pour castor oil over it.
2. Wear old clothes since the oil will stain your clothes
3. Place the castor oil cotton on the desired spot. Place a clean piece of cotton next to the oiled one
4. Place a non- toxic clear plastic over it.
5. Place your Earthwrappe, hot water bottle or heating pad next to the plastic. Keep it on for 60 minutes.
6. When finished, throw the cotton away. The cotton now contains the toxins from the affected area.
7. After the detox, I like to use Premier's Medi Body Bath. I go outside, weather permitting, and submerge my feet into the water to help speed up the detox process. I soak for 20 to 30 minutes.

Detox Works the Body's Natural Cleansing Process by

- Resting the organs through fasting.
- Stimulating the liver to drive toxins from the body.
- Promoting elimination through the intestines, kidneys and skin.
- Improving circulation of the blood.
- Refueling the body with healthy nutrients.

The body is always trying to get rid of toxins, always detoxifying through almost every organ. New research shows that almost every disease can be linked to toxicity. We live in such a toxic world, where everything around us like the air we breathe, the chemicals we clean with, the toxic chemicals used in gardening, the food we eat, what we put on our skin, and the toxins we drink.

So many things can add toxicity such as eating too much food or eating too much protein causing ammonia, also too much fat and sugar can kill off cells. As we age and the toxic load increases, it causes infection, inflammation and disease. At this point the only way we are going to heal is by using a good detox system.

Managing a detox system to reduce toxins before pregnancy is essential for giving you and your baby the best chance for maximum health. Cleaning our babies 9-month home will ensure the best possible environment for our baby to live and grow healthy.

"No Pain...No Gain" You May Have Detox Symptoms

Whether using a supplement program, introducing healthy foods, or using external detoxing and hopefully a combination of all three, you most likely will have detox symptoms. This is crucial to understand that the toxins are being released from your body. These symptoms usually last a few hours. However, this is proof that the toxins are starting to come out of your organs and into the bloodstream.

You May Experience Detox Symptoms Such as:

- Sick to your stomach
- Headache
- Extremely tired (hours to days)
- Pain in kidneys
- Diarrhea
- Swelling and retaining water

If you give up caffeine you can also experience detox symptoms, since you are ridding your body of toxins/drugs. The detox and/or supplement program may start to detox your body the same way. The more toxic, the more detoxing your body will need.

Here is a list of things that make the body more toxic:

- Taking medications
- Surgeries

- Eating junk foods (sugar, cakes, cookies)
- Poor digestion
- Poor dental health
- Hormonal imbalance

So let's recap…if you feel sick during a detox, you are removing toxins and that is a good thing (it will pass). Detox symptoms normally last a few hours. So, of course, it will depend on how sick you are. If you detox too quickly then we can always slow things down. If you have a terminal disease, then we would need to stay with the program and make your detox program an aggressive one. Remember it took years of toxicity to get you here, so you need to be patient as it will take some time to bring you back. Try to enjoy the journey, knowing a healthy you is in your future. Detoxification is a central component in long-term health.

Organs Responsible for Getting Rid of Toxin

The following organs will be especially critical in detoxing since they are the organs that are responsible for getting rid of toxins. It is important to show how our organs get rid of the toxins.

1. **Kidney**

   Symptoms: Buildup of waste products in the body that may cause weakness, shortness of breath, lethargy, and confusion.
   Disease: Kidney stones, kidney infection, and kidney failure.
   Body Function and Detox: Cleans the blood of toxins and urine.
   Detox Process: Drink filtered water to keep your kidneys working well.
   Supplements: use RenaVen, Mudpack to detox the kidneys, limit or eliminate medications under a doctor's care, especially antibiotics.

2. **Liver**

   Symptoms: Liver disease include weakness and fatigue, weight loss, nausea, vomiting, and yellow discoloration of the skin (jaundice).
   Disease: Cirrhosis occurs when normal liver cells are replaced by scar tissue.

Body Function: The main functions of the liver are to process nutrients from food, make bile, remove toxins from the body and build protein. The liver keeps toxins from damaging the body.
Detox Process: Limit alcohol, sugar and carbs. Do Liver Mudpack Detoxes.
Supplements: Premier Liver ND, Reishi, and HepatoVen.

3. **Lungs**
Symptoms: low oxygen level in blood, shortness of breath, bluish color on skin, lips and fingernails, confusion, sleepiness, loss of consciousness, and arrhythmias.
Disease: Bronchitis, COPD, Asthma, Pneumonia, Influenza, Lung Cancer, Sleep Apnea, Sudden Infant Death Syndrome, Tuberculosis, etc.
Body Function: The purpose of the lungs is to bring oxygen into the body and to remove carbon dioxide. Oxygen is a gas that provides us energy while carbon dioxide is a waste product or "exhaust" of the body.
Detox Process: Mudpack detox the lungs front and back. Supplements: Pneumo and Chem Detox. Eliminate all associations with all types of chemical and air toxins, and quit smoking!

4. **Lymphatic System**
Symptoms: Constantly sick or tired.
Disease: Lymphedema and Cancer.
Body Function: Your lymphatic system is comprised of your lymph nodes, spleen, thymus and vessels that carry fluids to protect your body from disease. They contain white blood cells that defend against disease.
Detox Process: Lymphatic massage and detox the lymph nodes.
Supplements: Medi Body Bath Soak, other foot soaks, sitting in infrared sauna

5. **Bladder**
Symptoms: Infections, burning sensation, urge to urinate, cloudy or bloody urine with strong foul odor, and bladder spasms. Cancer

- Pain in lower back, swelling in lower legs, growth in the pelvis, pain during urination, frequent urinary tract infections, and blood clots in urine.
Disease: Bladder Infections and Bladder Cancer.
Body Function: Urine is made in the kidneys, and travels down two tubes called ureters to the bladder. The bladder stores urine, allowing urination to be infrequent and voluntary.
Detox: The bladder works eliminating moisture accumulation in the body in the form of urine. It helps, along with the kidneys, to clean toxic buildup caused by the consumption of foods and liquids.
Supplements: RenaVen, UriVen.

6. **Colon**
Symptoms: Diarrhea, constipation, changes in stool consistency, blood in stool, weakness, fatigue, and unexplained weight loss.
Disease: Diverticulosis, Ulcerative Colitis, Irritable Bowel Syndrome, and Colon Cancer.
Body Function: Absorption of water and minerals, formation and elimination of feces, contains nearly 60 varieties of friendly bacteria to aid digestion, promote vital nutrient production, to maintain pH (acid-base) balance, and to prevent proliferation of harmful bacteria.
Detox: Eliminates toxins in the intestines. Colon Hydrotherapy and Juice Cleansing.
Supplements: HCL, Galectin, Premier Digest, and Digestase. Mudpack to detox the intestinal area.

This may be the last chapter, but it is the most important one. This includes any age; baby, toddler, teen, adult or older adult. I was 50 when I became ill and I was 58 when I healed from 18 diseases/disorders.... it is never too late.

Lisa's First Book - Why Can't I Lose Weight? Toxins

I was dying....I had 10 dead root canal teeth, hair loss, teeth and diseased nails along with 18 diseases/disorders. I also gained 50 pounds, mostly belly fat.

- I healed ....from **18 diseases**/disorders, mostly auto immune diseases:
- Hasimoto Thyroid
- Fibromyalgia
- Lyme Disease
- Type 2 Diabetes
- Adrenal Fatigue
- Arrhythmia
- Vertigo
- Epstein Barr
- IBS
- Celiac
- Migraines
- UTI's
- Candida
- RLS
- Depression
- Onion Allergy
- Gluten Intollerant
- Hair loss
- lost 40 pounds naturally.

What made me sick?....**Toxins**
How did I heal? .....**Detoxing**

"Ding Dong the Witch is Dead"

All the wicked witches in our fairy tales are dead; evil has died and goodness prevailed. Hansel and Gretel found their way home and decided not to eat cookies and candies no matter how good they looked. Cinderella married the Prince and she no longer had to clean with toxic chemicals or be insulted by toxic words; together they cleaned up all the toxins in the land. Snow White woke up and never ate another poison apple and helped children heal from the 7 deadly diseases of: Autism, ADHD, ADD, Asthma, SIDS, Diabetes and Obesity. Sleeping Beauty awoke and got rid of the fairy dust that had the entire Kingdom sleeping. She helped the world to wake up from eating, drinking, breathing, bathing, wearing, injecting and using harmful chemicals. Dorothy found her way home where she taught others how to grow healthy foods, "right in their own backyard." She learned from Oz, good foods will keep their **brains** sharp, their **hearts** healthy and give them the **courage** to stay away from the evil toxins.

"United we Stand, we will no Longer Fall"

Together we will build a stronger world with healthier foods and products, without the toxins. We all have a voice, and if we sing the same song and we sing it loud enough, we will have a hit record entitled "Healthy kids eat organic apples."

I pray that we will no longer LUST for unhealthy foods, or become GLUTTONS with excessive drinking, have a need for GREED to sell legal or illicet drugs, stop the LAZZINESS of sitting indoors, Get rid of the WRATH of anger and harsh words, will not ENVY to possess or steal from others and to have PRIDE in ourselves to spead love, kindness and good health throughout the world.

"And in the end we all lived happily ever after!"

LISA HEATHER TORBERT - BIOGRAPHY

Lisa gives new meaning to the words "been there done that," with her diverse array of talents, education, experiences, and achievements. Her ADHD worked to her advantage as an overachiever, conquering the business world by running a successful holistic health center in Dover, DE along with two other businesses. Her darker days, growing up in an Alcoholic family, molded her into the self-less giving careers as a Counselor, Hypnotherapist, & QRA Practitioner. She has overcome tragic lifelong sicknesses & diseases, healing from emotional illness and 18 different physical diseases. She not only holds a Masters in Counseling and is a Certified Addictions Counselor (CADC), she has earned the title of "addict" and understands emotional complexity. Her playful spirit enjoys guitar, keyboards, singing, songwriting and art. Her most satisfying gifts in life are the love from her family; husband, kids, parents, grandkids and her Shelties, Ziggy & Zeplin. She is determined to share the secrets to the healing power deep within our immune system. What distinguishes her from others is her personal branding, where she takes complicated and makes it easy, mixes facts and statistics with humor and pictures, all organized into a refreshing, innovative and interesting journey…a handbook to healing.

Books Published:
Why Can't I Lose Weight? Toxins
Healthy Kids Don't Eat Poison Apples

Youtube: https://www.youtube.com/watch?v=pE1rPjXBQgQ
Facebook: Lisa Heather Torbert Book
https://www.facebook.com/groups/1686131141662790/
Email: Heathersholistichealth@yahoo.com
Website: www.Heathersholistichealth.com

Helpful Sites and Companies

Facebook : "The Day Off Diet" by Dr OZ
https://www.facebook.com/groups/640748666066853/
Facebook: "Day Off Diet recipes To Share ☺ - https://www.facebook.com/groups/640748666066853/
Order Supplements: Premier Research Labs – supplements, energy devises - 800-370-3447
Order Foot soak: Jernigan Nutraceuticals – foot soak - 316-371-8485
Order Cats Claw: Raintree Formula 800-553-4657 - http://www.raintree.com/
Norwex cleaning products - https://norwex.biz/en_US/products
Holistic Dentistry – Julian Center - http://www.juliandentist.com/ (410) 964-3118

BIBLIOGRAPHY

Environmental Working Group. (November 23, 2009), Pollution In Minority Newborns, http://www.ewg.org/research/minority-cord-blood-report/bpa-and-other-cord-blood-pollutants

Institute for Optimal Health. (1996) http://www.ion.ac.uk/information/onarchives/infections

Infant formula warning: The poisoning of infants with formula products. (April 05, 2006), Alexis Black, thttp://www.naturalnews.com/019338_childrens_health_womens.html#ixzz3xKxC4mBm

US Food & Drug Administration (FDA). Bisphenol A (BPA): Use in Food Contact Application, (November 2014), http://www.fda.gov/food/ingredientspackaginglabeling/foodadditivesingredients/ucm064437.htm#overview

National Pesticide Information Center. http://npic.orst.edu/factsheets/cuso4gen.html npic@ace.orst.edu

Todays Parent, (Sep 2, 2015), Teresa Pitman
http://www.todaysparent.com/baby/baby-food/the-dos-and-donts-of-safe-formula-feeding/

Soybean Oil: One of the Most Harmful Ingredients in Processed Foods. (January 27, 2013) http://articles.mercola.com/sites/articles/archive/2013/01/27/soybean-oil.aspx

US Food & Drug Administration (FDA). (5/15/09) Vaccines, Blood & Biologics VAERS Overview, http://www.fda.gov/biologicsbloodvaccines/safetyavailability/reportaproblem/vaccineadverseevents/overview/default.htm

Centers for Disease (CDC) Control Vaccination Schedule. (2013). 414% Increase In Vaccines Given to U.S. Children, https://vactruth.com/history-of-vaccine-schedule/

Center for Disease Control and Prevention CDC. (Feb 22, 2011), Vaccines & Immunizations. Ingredients for Vaccines; Fact Sheet. http://www.cdc.gov/vaccines/vac-gen/additives.htm

Autism Society. (August 25, 2015), Facts and Statistics, http://www.autism-society.org/what-is/facts-and-statistics/

John F. McGowan, Ph.D. The Mathematics of Autism, (July 9, 2012), http://math-blog.com/2012/07/09/the-mathematics-of-autism/

U.S. Department of Health and Human Services, Basics A federal government Website http://www.vaccines.gov/basics/

Center for Disease Control (CDC). Vaccines and Immunizations, http://www.drugs.com/pro/flulaval.html drugs.com

Center for Disease Control (CDC). Vaccines http://www.cdc.gov/vaccines/parents/downloads/parent-ver-sch-0-6yrs.pdf

US Food & Drug Administration (FDA). US Study Reports Aluminum in Vaccines Poses Extremely Low Risk to Infants, (2/6/15), http://www.fda.gov/BiologicsBloodVaccines/ScienceResearch/ucm284520.htm

Natural Health 365. Why is neurotoxic aluminum in vaccines http://www.naturalhealth365.com/toxic_aluminum.html/

Neuroscience & Biobehavioral Reviews. William A. Banks, Abba J. Kastin. Aluminum-Induced neurotoxicity: Alterations in membrane function at the blood-brain barrier, http://www.sciencedirect.com/science/article/pii/S014976348980051X

Veggiesource, Sara Taylor. (June 5, 2013), Dairy Cows And Their Calves: When Mother Is Separated From Baby, http://www.vegsource.com/sarah-taylor/dairy-cows-and-their-calves-when-mother-is-separated-from-baby.html

Live Well Evansville. (2016), Why Immunize Our Children?, http://livewell-evansville.stmarys.org/why-immunize-our-children/#.VsTiEfk http://www.stmarys.org/rLIU

U.S. Health Care from a Global Perspective,(2013), http://www.commonwealthfund.org/publications/issue-briefs/2015/oct/us-health-care-from-a-global-perspective

Mother and Child Hospital. Preventable disease and the Vaccines that Prevent them, http://www.motherandchildhospital.in/vaccine-preventable-diseases-and-the-vaccines-that-prevent-them

Vactruit. History of Vaccine Schedule, https://vactruth.com/history-of-vaccine-schedule/

Center for Disease Control and Prevention (CDC), Prevalence of Obesity in the United States, 2009–2010, January 2012, Cynthia L. Ogden, Ph.D.; Margaret D. Carroll, M.S.P.H.; Brian K. Kit, M.D., M.P.H.; and Katherine M. Flegal, Ph.D.http://www.cdc.gov/nchs/data/databriefs/db82.htm

GMOs and the Deterioration of Health in the U.S. – A Comprehensive Guide. (June 11, 2013), https://johnniesblog.wordpress.com/2013/06/15/gmos-and-the-deterioration-of-health-in-the-u-s-a-comprehensive-guide/number-of-children-6-21-years-old-with-autism-06-11-2013/

Growth Opportunities in the Pharmaceuticals Sector, http://www.frost.com/prod/servlet/cpo/9459774

Center for Disease Control and Prevention. (December 2014), Mortality in the United States, 2013, http://www.cdc.gov/nchs/data/databriefs/db178.htm

Obesity in American Technology. (Feb. 16, 2016), https://obesity-documentary.rhcloud.com/obesity-in-america-technology.html

Dangerous Baby Toys, Kate Miller-Wilson. http://baby.lovetoknow.com/wiki/Dangerous_Baby_Toys

One Step Ahead. "How to Choose the Best Baby Toys", (2016), http://www.onestepahead.com/articles/buying-for-children/choose-the-best-baby-toys

USA TODAY. Liz Szabo, "Diabetes rates skyrocket in kids and teens", (May 3, 2014), http://www.usatoday.com/story/news/nation/2014/05/03/diabetes-rises-in-kids/8604213/

US Food & Drug Administration (FDA). "Mortality in the United States", (2014), http://www.cdc.gov/nchs/data/databriefs/db229.htm

The International Council for Truth in Medicine. "Death by Medicine: How Medical Errors and Prescription Drugs Kill 1 Million People a Year" http://www.theictm.org/death-by-medicine-how-medical-errors-and-prescription-drugs-kill-1-million-people-a-year#.Vw1Nl_krLIU

American Psychiatric Association. (1994), "Diagnostic and statistical manual of mental disorders (4th ed)"

CBS Health Watch. (2000) "Educate Before You Medicate Your Kids" www.CBSHealthWatch.com

VillageandallHealth. (2000) "Alternative Parenting", www.alternativeparenting.com/health/ADD

Special Education Degrees. "Colors to Die", http://www.special-education-degree.net/food-dyes/

National Sleep Foundation. "ADHD and Sleep", https://sleepfoundation.org/sleep-disorders-problems/adhd-and-sleep

Additude Magazine. "Game On: 10 Best Sports for Kids with ADHD or Learning Disabilities", http://www.additudemag.com/slideshow/104/slide-10.html.

Brain Balance Center. "Studies shows exercise helps kids with ADHD", http://www.brainbalancecenters.com/blog/2014/10/studies-show-exercise-helps-adhd-kids/

Psychiatry Research 220(1-2). (November 2014), https://www.researchgate.net/publication/262841497_Blood_manganese_levels_in_relation_to_comorbid_behavioral_and_emotional_problems_in_children_with_attention-deficithyperactivity_disorder

Body Unburdened. "How food is responsible for behavioral issues in children," (June 30, 2013), http://bodyunburdened.com/food-dye-behavioral-issues-children/

Eric H. Chudler. "The Blood Brain Barrier ("Keep Out")", (2015), https://faculty.washington.edu/chudler/bbb.html

Phyllis A. Balch. "Prescription for Nutritional Healing," Sulfer Foods

Autism Society. "Facts and Statistics" http://www.autism-society.org/what-is/facts-and-statistics/

National Institutes of Health. (December 30, 2015), "Distribution and Predictors of Pesticides in the Umbilical Cord Blood of Chinese Newborns US National Library of Medicine" http://www.ncbi.nlm.nih.gov/pmc/articles/PMC4730485/

National Institutes of Health. (February, 4, 2016), "Natural Product-Derived Treatments for Attention-Deficit/Hyperactivity Disorder: Safety, Efficacy, and Therapeutic Potential of Combination Therapy", http://www.ncbi.nlm.nih.gov/pmc/articles/PMC4757677/

SAMHSA. (2013), "Center for Behavioral Health Statistics and Quality, National Survey on Drug Use and Health", https://www.google.com/search?q=statistics+for+adhd+add+charts+2014&newwindow=1&espv=2&biw=1517&bih=692&source=lnms&tbm=isch&sa=X&ved=0ahUKEwj5hPKm6anMAhUMaz4KHdN8BG8Q_AUICCgD&dpr=0.9#imgrc=pn7LQOXgh-AOPM%3A:

ADHD/ADD: The War On Children. Reasons for Drug-Related Emergency Department (ED) Visits, by Year: 2004 to 2011", https://www.google.com/search?q=statistics+for+adhd+add+charts+2014&newwindow=1&espv=2&biw=1517&bih=692&source=lnms&tbm=isch&sa=X&ved=0ahUKEwj5hPKm6anMAhUMaz4KHdN8BG8Q_AUICCgD&dpr=0.9#newwindow=1&tbm=isch&q=statistics+for+adhd+add+charts+years+&imgrc=jmOP4wzHpoaqwM%3A

Center for Disease Center (CDC.) "New Data: Medication and Behavior Treatment, Attention-Deficit / Hyperactivity Disorder (ADHD)"

Shannon Hutton. (Jun 25, 2013), "Helping Visual Learners Succeed" http://www.education.com/magazine/article/Helping_Visual_Learners/

Warner Bros. Cartoons. (1948 and 1966), The Road Runner Show Wile E. Coyote, The Road Runner lyrics from the Looney Tunes and Merrie Melodies

Amanda Chan. (April 01, 2011), " live Science… 3 Ways Technology Affects Your Eyes", http://www.livescience.com/35579-3-ways-technology-affects-eyes.html

"Internet Overuse Could Cause Structural Brain Damage", (January, 14, 2012), http://www.gmanetwork.com/news/story/244614/scitech/science/internet-overuse-can-damage-brain-china-researchers

Inside Edition. "Tucking Cell Phone in Bra May be Connected to Breast Cancer", (June 11, 2013), http://www.insideedition.com/headlines/6477-tucking-cell-phone-in-bra-may-be-connected-to-breast-cancer

Nipun. (October 19, 2015), "Difference Between Ionizing and Nonionizing Radiation", Nipun http://pediaa.com/difference-between-ionizing-and-nonionizing-radiation/

Bloomize. "Magnetic Stuff Around the House," http://www.bloomize.com/magnetic-stuff-around-the-house/

Nasa. "Sources of Gama Ray," http://missionscience.nasa.gov/ems/12_gammarays.html

"Learn About The Types of Electromagnetic Radiation So You Can Protect and Improve Your Health," http://www.best-emf-health.com/types-of-electromagnetic-radiation.html

"Electromagnetic Fields (EMF) and Radio Frequency (RF) Radiation Indoor Environmental Technologies," http://www.ietbuildinghealth.com/electromagnetic-inspections.htm

"Whats wrong with Strict Parenting? Whats wrong with Permissive Parenting?" http://www.ahaparenting.com/parenting-tools/positive-discipline/permissive-parenting

National Institute of Health (NIH), (Jan 2004), " Effective discipline for children, Pediatric Child Care," http://www.ncbi.nlm.nih.gov/pmc/articles/PMC2719514/

Parents. "When Does Discipline Begin?" http://www.parents.com/baby/development/behavioral/when-does-discipline-begin1/

Center for Disease Control (CDC). "Reducing Chemical Accidents Involving Pesticides, Mercury, ATSDR Cleaning Products, and Science Labs in Schools," http://www.atsdr.cdc.gov/ntsip/docs/Reducing_Chemicals_in_Schools.pdf

Center for Disease Control (CDC). "Public Health Statement -Agency for Toxic Substances," http://www.atsdr.cdc.gov/toxprofiles/tp111-c1.pdf

Center for Disease Control (CDC). "2016 Recommended Immunizations for Birth Through 6 Years Old", http://www.cdc.gov/vaccines/parents/downloads/parent-ver-sch-0-6yrs.pdf

US Department of health and social services. "Household product database," https://hpd.nlm.nih.gov/cgi-bin/household/search?tbl=TblChemicals&queryx=50-00-0

Marilee Nelson. (June 11, 2015), "Common Household Chemicals | Phthalates: 19 Surprising Sources," https://branchbasics.com/blog/2015/06/common-household-chemicals-phthalates-19-surprising-sources/

Matt Tomasino. (July 24, 2013) "PEVA/EVA Plastic - Is it really green, or just a wash?" http://www.greenhome.com/blog/pevaeva-plastic-is-it-really-green-or-just-a-wash

Jessie Sholl. (October 2011), "8 Hidden toxins Whats lurking in your Cleaning Products?" https://experiencelife.com/article/8-hidden-toxins-whats-lurking-in-your-cleaning-products/

Awesome Beginning Children. "The Harmful Chemicals in Disposable Diapers" http://awesomebeginnings4children.com/the-harmful-chemicals-in-disposable-diapers/

Green America. (February 2003), "Solving the Diaper Dilemma." http://www.greenamerica.org/livinggreen/diapers.cfm

Holly Rhodes. Fluff Love University. "Washing Your Diapers In Plant-based or Free and Clear Detergents," http://www.fluffloveuniversity.com/how-to-wash-cloth-diapers/washing-your-diapers-in-plant-based-or-free-and-clear-detergents/

Eco Babysteps. Attached Mama. (April 30, 2013), "Hemp vs Bamboo Rayon for Cloth Diapers," http://www.ecobabysteps.com/2013/04/30/hemp-vs-bamboo-rayon-for-cloth-diapers/

"Non Toxic Revolution" (February 26, 2013), http://nontoxicrevolution.org/blog/the-diaper-dilemma-lowdown-best-non-toxic-diaper-options-for-your-baby/#.VyqHroQrLIU

Center for Disease Control (CDC). "Insufficient Sleep Is a Public Health Problem," http://www.cdc.gov/features/dssleep/

National Institute of Health (NIH). "What Are the Signs and Symptoms of Problem Sleepiness?" http://www.nhlbi.nih.gov/health/health-topics/topics/sdd/signs

Better Health. "Conditions and Treatments," https://www.betterhealth.vic.gov.au/health/conditionsandtreatments/sleep-deprivation

Denise Fields and Ari Brown, MD. Meredith Corporation. Lucile Packard Children's Hospital at Stanford University; National Sleep Foundation, Baby 411 and Toddler 411. (2008), "How Much Sleep Does Your Child Need?" http://www.parents.com/baby/sleep/basics/age-by-age-guide/

WebMD Medical Reference. "What Are REM and Non-REM Sleep?" http://www.webmd.com/sleep-disorders/guide/sleep-101

Rapid eye movement sleep. https://en.wikipedia.org/wiki/Rapid_eye_movement_sleep

National Institute of Health (NIH). "What Are the Signs and Symptoms of Sleep Apnea?" https://www.nhlbi.nih.gov/health/health-topics/topics/sleepapnea/signs

Whitney Jefferson. (April, 23, 2012), "27 Yoga Positions Demonstrated By Animals," https://www.buzzfeed.com/whitneyjefferson/the-animal-guide-to-yoga?utm_term=.xmYjAxKrp0#.vd20GwY4Zq

Lyndee Fletcher/Movie Guide. (10/15/2015), "14 Mass Murders Linked to Violent Video Games" http://www.charismanews.com/culture/52651-14-mass-murders-linked-to-violent-video-games

"Snuggle science: Why cuddling is good for your health," http://fusion.net/story/50195/cuddling-is-good-for-your-health/ HUG IT OUT 2/17/15 6:22 PM

Kelly Rober, I Love to Know Health. "Top Ten Relaxation Techniques for Children" http://stress.lovetoknow.com/Top_Ten_Relaxation_Techniques_Children

Mr. Breakfast. "All Breakfast all the Time," http://www.mrbreakfast.com/list.asp?id=2

Deena Shanke. (2014), "23 Healthy And Easy Breakfasts Your Kids Will Love," https://www.buzzfeed.com/deenashanker/healthy-easy-breakfasts-your-kids-will-love?utm_term=.hiLXbjgDl8#.dvBpMPXRG2

Carol Kicinski. (Septeber 15, 2013) "Simply Gluten Free Gluten Free Mexican Mini Quiches Recipe," https://simplygluten-free.com/blog/2013/09/gluten-free-mexican-mini-quiches-recipe.html

Mayo Clinci. "Healthy Lifestyle Infant and toddler health," http://www.mayoclinic.org/healthy-lifestyle/infant-and-toddler-health/in-depth/breast-milk-storage/art-20046350?pg=2

Wholesome Baby Food Momtastic. "Sample Baby Food Menu for Babies (4) 6-8 months old," http://wholesomebabyfood.momtastic.com/babymenua.htm, and http://wholesomebabyfood.momtastic.com/babymenua.htm#t41G5pYpdbVsa5w3.99

Wellness Mama. "How to Get Kids to Eat Healthy Food," http://wellness-mama.com/1063/guide-to-feeding-healthy-kids/

Environmental Working Group. (July, 14, 2005), "Body Burden: The Pollution in Newborns: A Benchmark Investigation of Industrial." http://www.ewg.org/research/body-burden-pollution-newborns

Autism Society. (July 15, 2015), "Causes" http://www.autism-society.org/what-is/causes/

Autism Speaks. "Medicines for Treating Autism's Core Symptoms" https://www.autismspeaks.org/what-autism/treatment/medicines-treating-core-symptoms

Autism Science Foundation. "What is Autism?" http://autismsciencefoundation.org/what-is-autism/

WEbmed. "Childrens Vaccines," http://www.webmd.com/children/vaccines/features/vaccine-linked-to-autism

Lisa Joyce Goes. (2013), 30 Scientific Studies Showing the Link between Vaccines and Autism. http://healthimpactnews.com/2013/30-scientific-studies-showing-the-link-between-vaccines-and-autism/#sthash.D8WOGQdF.dpuf

Autism Speaks. "Family Grant Opportunities" https://www.autismspeaks.org/family-services/resource-library/family-grant-opportunities

Laurie Tarkan. (March 29, 2016), "Why Robert De Niro Promoted -- then Pulled -- Anti-Vaccine Documentary," http://fortune.com/2016/03/29/robert-de-niro-anti-vaccine-documentary/

Center for Disease Center (CDC). "Asthma Attacks Among Persons with Current Asthma — United States, 2001–2010", (Nov. 22, 2013), http://www.cdc.gov/mmwr/preview/mmwrhtml/su6203a16.htm?s_cid=su6203a16_e

National Institute of Health (NIH). "How Can Asthma be Prevented", https://www.nhlbi.nih.gov/health/health-topics/topics/asthma/prevention

Home Remedies.com. "Home Remedies for Asthma," http://www.top10homeremedies.com/home-remedies/home-remedies-for-asthma.html

Beyond Pesticides. "Products Containing Triclosan," http://www.beyondpesticides.org/programs/antibacterials/triclosan/products-containing-triclosan

Environmental Working Group (EWG) Sites

https://www.ewg.org/skindeep/browse.php?category=nail_polish&&showmore=products&start=10

https://www.ewg.org/skindeep/browse/baby+wipes/

https://www.ewg.org/skindeep/search.php?query=baby+wash

https://www.ewg.org/skindeep/search.php?query=toothpaste

https://www.ewg.org/skindeep/search.php?query=soap

https://www.ewg.org/skindeep/search.php?query=skin+moisturizers

https://www.ewg.org/skindeep/search.php?query=sunscreen

http://www.ewg.org/2015sunscreen/report/the-trouble-with-sunscreen-chemicals/

http://www.ewg.org/skindeep/search.php?query=shampoo

http://www.ewg.org/skindeep/search.php?query=hair+spray

https://www.ewg.org/skindeep/product/173725/KMS_California_Hairstay_Spray%2C_Maximum_Hold_%282008_formulation%29/

http://www.ewg.org/2015sunscreen/report/the-trouble-with-sunscren-chemicals/

http://www.ewg.org/hair-straighteners/our-report/hair-straighteners-that-hide-formaldehyde/

US Food and Drug Administration (FDA). "Phthalates," http://www.fda.gov/Cosmetics/ProductsIngredients/Ingredients/ucm128250.htm

US Food and Drug Administration (FDA). "For Consumers: Seven Things Pregnant Women and Parents Need to Know About Arsenic in Rice and Rice Cereal," http://www.fda.gov/forconsumers/consumerupdates/ucm493677.htm

Simply Vegan 5th Edition, Reed Mangels, PhD, "Iron in the Vegan Diet," http://www.vrg.org/nutrition/iron.php

Non Dairy Calcium Rich Foods. https://www.google.com/search?q=high+calcium+in+non+dairy+list&newwindow=1&espv=2&biw=1517&bih=741&source=lnms&tbm=isch&sa=X&ved=0ahUKEwjHspnvkdfMAhWD8j4KHR3JAZ4Q_AUICCgD&dpr=0.9#imgrc=2ChzgLcp-iznrM%3A

National Institute of Health (NIH), Warnock DW1, Delves HT, Campell CK, Croudace IW, Davey KG, Johnson EM, Sieniawska C. (1995), "Toxic gas generation from plastic mattresses and sudden infant death syndrome." http://www.ncbi.nlm.nih.gov/pubmed/7491046

National Institute of Health (NIH) Murrell TG1, Murrell WG, Lindsay JA., "Sudden infant death syndrome (SIDS): are common bacterial toxins responsible, and do they have a vaccine potential?" http://www.ncbi.nlm.nih.gov/pubmed/8178560

Dr. Oz, Dr. Majid Fotuhi. (5/30/2012), "The Brain Diet," http://www.doctoroz.com/article/brain-diet

US Food and Drug Administration (FDA). "Thimerosal in Vaccines," http://www.fda.gov/biologicsbloodvaccines/safetyavailability/vaccinesafety/ucm096228.htm

Parents Magazine, Kristen Finello. "Chickenpox Parties," http://www.parents.com/health/vaccines/chicken-pox/chickenpox-parties/

Charts

Vactruth. "Vaccine Schedule", https://vactruth.com/history-of-vaccine-schedule/

The Commonwealth Fund. "US Healthcare from a Global Perspective", http://www.commonwealthfund.org/publications/issue-briefs/2015/oct/us-health-care-from-a-global-perspective

NationalInstituteofHealth(NIH)."PrinciplesofAdolescentSubstanceUseDisorder Treatment: A Research-Based Guide" https://www.drugabuse.gov/publications/principles-adolescent-substance-use-disorder-treatment-research-based-guide/introduction

Workout Austraila. "Dairy Free Calcium Food Sources", http://www.workoutaustralia.com.au/news/dairy-free-calcium-food-sources

National Institute of Health (NIH). "Mortality in the US 2012" http://www.cdc.gov/nchs/products/databriefs/db168.htm

Center for Disease Center (CDC). "International Comparisons of Infant Mortality and Related Factors: United States and Europe 2010", http://www.cdc.gov/nchs/data/nvsr/nvsr63/nvsr63_05.pdf

Center for Disease Center (CDC). (December 2015), "Mortality in the United States, 2014" http://www.cdc.gov/nchs/products/databriefs/db229.htm

US National Ambulatory Medical Care Survey (NAMCS) "The Age of ADHD", https://www.google.com/search?q=rate+of+office+based+visits+adhd&sou

rce=lnms&tbm=isch&sa=X&ved=0ahUKEwjQ_sOg2oLNAhUK6yYKHVIwD UEQ_AUICCgC&biw=1252&bih=554#imgrc=jmOP4wzHpoaqwM%3A

Vanderbilt Assessment Scale http://www.myadhd.com/vanderbiltparent6175.html

Center for Disease Center (CDC). "Number of Children with Asthma". http://www.cdc.gov/media/releases/2014/p0327-autism-spectrum-disorder.html

Socioecohistory. "Vaccines and Autism" https://socioecohistory.wordpress.com/2015/03/07/

https://www.google.com/search?q=moans+stones+groans+and+bones&source=lnms&tbm=isch&sa=X&ved=0ahUKEwiftvPo_J7NAhWCpR4KHUsRDE0Q_AUICSgC&biw=1252&bih=554#tbm=isch&q=hormone+with+human+body+chart&imgrc=v75AiGXNsMArOM%3A

YouTube Videos

Youtube videos on Vaxxed featuring Robert Deniro

https://www.youtube.com/watch?v=EdCU2DfMBpU
https://www.youtube.com/watch?v=FJ7iPn39i08

www.ingramcontent.com/pod-product-compliance
Lightning Source LLC
Chambersburg PA
CBHW071329280526
45787CB00001B/39
9781533422668